Ketogenic Solutions

Finally Lose the Weight and Truly Feel Great

Heather Parker

Copyright © 2016

Become a Nourish, Grow & Thrive member (3 month, 6 month, and on-going memberships available) and receive monthly meal plans and shopping lists, discounted coaching packages, and access to a supportive private Facebook group.

Join Heather at:
ItStartsWithTheFood.com

Legal Disclaimer

To You, From Me

When I sat down at my computer in April of 2015, I had no idea that I would be writing for an audience bigger than the five people who had reached out to me for help. I went through profound changes in my life, never expecting these changes to be inspirational or the catalyst for others to do the same.

Within a few days of each other, I had five different people approach me, desperate for a better solution. A few came to me because of weight issues; others because they wanted health on their own terms… all of them got what they came for, which was a surprise only to them. It was not a surprise to me. I already knew that weight is a symptom of a lack of health.

This was the beginning of my OG's, my Original Group. Over a period of a few months, that group grew. People started to take notice of the changes happening to those five ladies.

Word started to spread and my phone started to ring. When I realized there were more people out there that could benefit from my struggles and experiences, a fire lit within me. My purpose and passion became obvious.

Without the commitment to change from my OG's, this book and everything that came along with it would not have happened. Their willingness to trust me and to trust the process kept me in the game. Through their successes and stumbles, I've been here because they kept showing up.

My husband Danny and sister Marlo, better known as my Wise Counsel, have given me sage advice on more than one occasion. I couldn't ask for two better people to have in my corner. You guys are truly my best friends and biggest cheerleaders.

Of course, I can't forget my kids. I went from a full-time mom and homeschool teacher to a hermit typing away madly in my bedroom. Your patience and help around the house didn't go unnoticed. Thank you for letting me do my thing.

XOXO
Heather

Table of Contents

Chapter 1: How I Got Here

Chapter 1: HOW I GOT HERE

My journey started many years ago, probably when I first overheard the word "chubby" while the adults were talking about me. It was the first time I became aware of my body and it was completely unfair because I was just about to go through puberty. I now know as an adult that puberty begins with weight gain, but nobody told that to the "chubby" 10 year old me. From that moment on, my life revolved around weight and body image.

I have spent most of my entire life sick. And not just a little sick, but the type of sick that doctors are mystified by. That kid that was always missing school due to one illness or the other… yeah, that was me. There was a good chance that, on any given day, I would be on antibiotics.

I had the chicken pox. Twice. I developed shingles at 13. I had my first ulcer by 15, my first kidney infection at 17, and first colonoscopy at 21. Yup, I was a keeper.

In my teens, I developed chronic strep throat until my tonsils were removed at the age of 16. That would be the first of 14 surgeries over a span of 25 years.

If there was an award for most illnesses by the age of 21, I could have won it.

I was diagnosed with GERD (Gastroesophageal reflux disease) at 21, and IBS and Fibromyalgia in my mid-20s. "Sick" was my normal, and it got to the point that I had no idea what healthy looked or felt like.

My normal got a whole lot worse 7 years ago. I started having huge blood-pressure swings, my heart rate would stay over 100, spiking into the 160s even in my sleep; I had headaches, and edema that was so severe that I would retain 15-20 pounds of water in a matter of days. I bounced around from one specialist to the other: multiple cardiologists, an endocrinologist, a nephrologist (what's that?! Who knows, but I saw one), an internal medicine specialist, an infectious disease doctor, you name it, they all saw me.

None had answers and some even suggested taking drastic measures without even knowing if it would make a difference. I ended up walking away with my medicine cabinets full of pills to treat the symptoms, but no cause in sight.

It was no way to live.

I had already seen the power of what the right food could do. My nephew had been brought back from the grips of an autistic diagnosis through proper nutrition and I thought maybe the answer for me might be there, too.

I started making changes in my diet, beginning with removing gluten and swapping out conventional meats and produce with organic versions. I started seeing improvements.

I had a long way to go and many more changes to make before I realized true health. It took removing all varieties of processed foods, letting go of my reliance on restaurants, cooking for myself, and switching to using Himalayan pink salt instead of the typical table salt, to create the most drastic change.

My body responded to real food unlike any medicine I had ever taken. I removed sugars, grains, and most fruit. My diet now is heavy in non-starchy vegetables, organic and preferably locally grown, pasture-raised chicken and eggs, raw grass-fed cheese, grass-fed and finished beef, wild-caught salmon, raw organic nuts (soaked and sprouted whenever possible), lots of the good saturated fats like coconut oil and avocados, and unpasteurized dairy when I can get it.

I try to buy most of my food from small stores that deal directly with the farmers so I have peace of mind with the food I bring into my house.

Even though it started off as a journey to weight loss, it ended in a true space of wellbeing for me. The weight loss was just a bonus. Now that I know what healthy feels like, I also know how my body reacts whenever I deviate from this lifestyle. When I was always sick, it was impossible for me to gauge how food affected me. Now I know better.

The First Year

In the first 45 years of my life, I was every size from a 0 to a 14 and two things never changed: 1) I was chronically ill and 2) I was chronically unhappy with my body. I look back at pictures of a much younger version of myself and I just want to put my arms around that me and let her know we do eventually figure it all out.

The last three years have been eye-opening and liberating. I knew that eating was a big part of my health so that first year I cut out gluten. I went organic. And I limited my fast food intake to Chipotle or Burgerfi. I watched my family losing weight and having all sorts of great health side effects, yet I just felt defeated and tired. I thought I was really getting a raw deal: I was doing all of the work, being diligent about what I was eating, and I got nothing, nada, zip.

I was still sick more days than not and still heavy. I would get on the scale of misery and hold my breath until the digital numbers appeared. So many days ruined all because I got on the scale that morning. It set the tone for my day, especially if I was feeling optimistic about what would be revealed on the scale. If I had dropped a pound or two, I let that make it a great day.

If I gained a pound or two, that was a totally different story. I beat myself up. I would dissect every little thing I ate the day before and try to reconcile any exercise I did to negate any of the calories I had eaten throughout the day. None of it made any sense. It was the first time in my life I thought that maybe after 40, this was it, I wasn't going to ever see a size 8, let alone a 0 (!). Worse, I worried that I was destined to be a sickly senior citizen.

The Second Year: Full of Disappointment

The second year, my husband and I had our 15th anniversary and I booked us a spectacular trip to Cancun to renew our vows. I booked the trip in March and the trip was at the end of September.

In the interim, I spent 6 days a week at the gym. I would do an hour of cardio and another 45 minutes on weights. I mixed in a lot of cycling, yoga, Pilates, and Zumba classes too.

Sometimes, I even did 2 classes a day. I was definitely healthier than I had ever been, but I became extremely frustrated during those months. I never had any significant losses on the scale. I started at 155 and the lowest I ever hit during that frenetic time was 148.

We all carry weight differently, but at 5'3, I carried it everywhere. My face has always been my tell - in more than one way. It is the first place I gain and lose weight, which was why I hated pictures of myself. All I could see when I would look at myself was that chubby girl with the round face.

During those months at the gym, I did start to feel better about myself because, at the very least, my fat wasn't quite as jiggly. We went on our trip and got beautiful pictures taken of my husband and myself renewing our vows. We received the pictures in the mail after we got back from Mexico and that was it for me: I was done killing myself in the gym because obviously, it wasn't making any difference in my weight.

What I imagined the pictures looking like versus what I saw made me so sad.

I came to terms with the fact that having had a full hysterectomy at 41, I was never going to be the 40-something that looks 'amazing for her age'. I slowly started eating more sugar, gluten-free packaged foods, carbs of all shapes and sizes, and soon became a shape and a size beyond where I had been before.

During those months, I became sickly again. I seemed to be sick with some kind of virus or bug all of the time. I don't think I ever got up in the morning feeling rested and ready to attack the day.

Rock Bottom

In May of 2014, everything came to a head. I had topped out at 164 pounds, which was 10 pounds more than I was at the end of both of my pregnancies, and I felt like an old woman.

Summer comes early here in Florida and none of my weather-appropriate clothes fit. As much as I hated it, I had to go to Target to find clothes I could wear for running errands. I ended up coming home with my first and last pair of size 14 shorts.

This was a major turning point.

I was miserable every time I went into my closet to try to find something other than yoga pants to wear. Forget about going out or anything else that would force me to try on half my wardrobe just to put on something that didn't make me look homeless.

In April, I booked my husband and I another trip to Mexico for our anniversary in October. Not only did I not fit into my clothes, but I was going to have to be in a bathing suit in less than five months. I also had a trip to Vegas in June and a wedding to attend at the end of May.

I knew things had to change.

Shortly after booking that trip to Mexico, I tried a lean protein/low-fat diet. It was a total failure and only lasted for four days. The good that came out of this was that I was introduced to something I'd never heard of called the "ketogenic concept." I felt that I had failed miserably on an all lean protein diet, but I should say the all lean protein diet failed me.

I needed answers so I did quite a bit of reading and researching on the ketogenic diet. I had done every other diet in the past including Primal, Paleo, Atkins, low-fat/low-calorie, grapefruit, cayenne pepper/honey water... after the four-day fiasco, I wasn't ready to jump into another diet but I also hadn't dismissed it entirely.

It took hitting rock bottom for me to go all in, this one last time.

I became convinced that we had all been lied to about fats and knew wheat - whole or otherwise - wasn't good for our bodies. I read *Wheat Belly*, watched documentaries like *Food Inc.*, and spent hours doing research on the Internet, so I was primed for a new way of life.

I just had to hit a bottom big enough for me to want to try one more time.

I read about the health and weight loss benefits with the ketogenic lifestyle (I have a hard time calling it a diet), so I figured it was at least worth attempting. I can't say I was convinced it was going to work but I also figured it couldn't hurt.

I had no idea that I was about to embark on a journey that would not only change my life, but would potentially change the lives of so many around me.

Victory at Last

That was in May 2014, and my life has transformed into so much more than I could have ever hoped for.

On the Ketogenic diet, I immediately started losing weight. I never had any big drops on the scale, but I was consistently losing 1-2 pounds a week from the start. After the first month, I realized I wasn't feeling sick anymore. I was more active, getting more done in a day, not feeling rundown or tired, and even looking forward to participating in my life.

The scale no longer scared me - I weighed myself every day and it wasn't depressing! In fact, the scale was reflecting the changes I was seeing in my body. I really wish I had taken my measurements when I first started because I could feel my body shrinking. It was about so much more than just losing weight.

I was becoming a fat burner. From day to day, it seemed as though I was losing size faster than the scale was showing.

Within 8 months of starting, I was wearing a size 0-2 (depending on where I buy the clothes.) I lost 8 inches in my waist, 5 inches in my thighs, down 3 inches in my arms, and went from a 36G bra size to a 34D. I have dropped a total of 50 pounds and am thrilled to be 114-117 pounds on any given day. (A fluctuation of 3-4 pounds is normal for me at any weight and is usually affected by what I have eaten the previous day or two.) Eating out, even the healthiest choices, always seem to cause a 2 pound temporary gain on the scale.

After two days, I'm back to where I should be.

Over this time period I regained my health. Now I am healthier than I have ever been in my entire life. When I go to the gym to do Pilates or Yoga, it's because I want to, not because I'm desperately trying to work off the pounds.

During the first year, I incorporated so many things into my lifestyle. I changed what I ate, when I ate it, and added meditation into my routine. I found my joy again. I was at peace with myself and the world around me. I don't think weight equates to happiness but I do know that not hating myself for being sick, tired, and fat really helps the happy. I felt empowered knowing the food I choose to put in my body helps me continue to be healthy.

I have taken my health back. I have control over my weight. I have my happy.

And now I want the same for you, too.

Fear and Desperation

As I have moved along this new path, I have heard one note consistently: fear.

It sounds like this: "I'm scared to actually hope this could be the answer to my struggles."

I promise you, you would not be here if you'd been successful doing anything else! I didn't get here because life was good. I got here out of desperation and didn't dare to hope it might actually work.

But I really had no other choice. I was done with being sick, tired, and fat.

Trust the process, give yourself a chance to succeed. If you follow my lead, I will provide you with all that you need to overcome any hurdles. Together, we can look at what you're doing, or not doing in some cases, to see what can be tweaked or adjusted.

Everyone is different, so you may need to modify from the precise path I took. The good news is that the major milestones will be very similar, so my experience can help you.

Ready?

Let's get started.

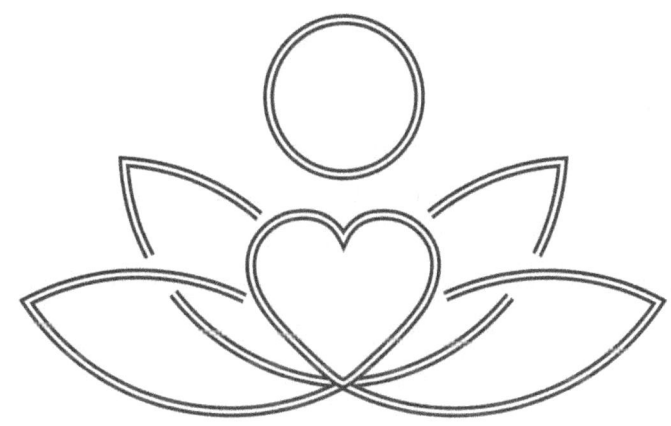

Chapter 2: Ketogenics and Ketosis

Chapter 2: KETOGENICS AND KETOSIS

I Inhaled the Cream Cheese

Until May 2014, I had never heard of the ketogenic diet. As I recounted in the previous chapter, I found out about it by accident (okay, so I don't really believe in accidents) after trying an all lean protein diet a girlfriend of mine had great success with.

I watched her transform her body over the period of a year through working out like a maniac and eating a diet high in lean protein and extremely low in fat. I wasn't willing to become part of the Crossfit craze - I still held some deep resentment towards my gym - but I was down with trying the lean protein thing.

I stocked up my fridge with turkey breasts, chicken breasts, lean meats in every shape and flavor, and the standard vegetables. I lasted a whopping four days before I became too sick to continue.

I found myself starving despite my plate full of chicken breasts. The thought of trying to cram another piece of turkey into my mouth made me nauseous. I had a headache for 2 straight days and felt like I was dying. I remember looking into the refrigerator and seeing a package of cream cheese and before I knew it, I grabbed a spoon and the cream cheese and proceeded to polish off half the container.

My headache disappeared almost instantly and the feeling of starvation vanished, as well. It happened so quickly, it caused me to drop everything to do some investigating. I went straight to my computer to see if I could figure out why it worked.

After spending a few minutes Googling different words, I came across an article that referenced something called "Rabbit Starvation".

This is a form of malnutrition caused by too much protein and not enough fat. It was something from which the Native Americans would suffer during long winters when they had nothing but rabbit to eat. Rabbit is an extremely lean meat and did not provide them with enough of the fat they needed.

The symptoms of this form of malnutrition include diarrhea, headache, fatigue, low blood pressure and a hunger that can only be satisfied with the addition of fat into the diet.

EUREKA!!! I had found my answer.
I started reading more information on this website, which happened to be about the ketogenic diet. This led me to other websites with even more information. I have no doubt that if I had not gone down the rabbit hole (ha!) with the lean protein diet, it may not have resonated with me as much as it did.

I had first-hand experience with how my body responded to a lack of fat. I inhaled half a container of cream cheese. This was enough for me to explore the diet further.

Ketogenics 101

As far back as 500 BC, there have been diets created to treat epilepsy by tricking the metabolism into thinking it's in a fasting state. The ancient Greeks were the first to observe how fasting would lessen the frequency and severity of seizures. In the early 1920s, this information was used to create the Ketogenic diet, specifically for treating seizures.

It was effective and commonly prescribed for epileptics until the introduction of anti-seizure medications and then pharmaceuticals became the standard treatment. Over the past 15 years, the Ketogenic diet has made a comeback for the treatment of epilepsy, especially in children. Quite a few of the anti-seizure medications have side-effects and can even become ineffective after long-term use.

The ketogenic diet consists of mostly fats, some proteins, low-carbs and lots of non-starchy vegetables. The ratio is generally 75% fats, 20% proteins, 5% carbs. The diet eliminates things like grains of all kinds including rice, bread, pasta, flour, oats, wheat, grits and tortilla chips, sugar, processed food, potatoes (other than the rare sweet potato), and limits real food higher in carbs. Those can be a little trickier to identify.

Reading labels is the best way to know if what you're eating is high in carbs.

The whole premise behind this way of eating is to put the body into a state of ketosis by lowering carb intake and allowing for moderate protein consumption. Most of us don't need large amounts of protein (found this out the hard way) so what we don't use will be turned into carbs for our bodies to then convert into glucose. That's why eating more protein isn't necessarily a good thing when trying to achieve a state of ketosis.

There are really two types of carbs; high-glycemic index carbs and low-glycemic index carbs. The difference between the two is the impact each has on our blood sugar.

When we eat things like breads, pasta or sugar, it causes our blood sugar levels to rise quickly. That, in turn, causes the body to produce a lot of insulin to counteract the sugar flooding the body.
When we eat foods that fall in the low-glycemic index range, there is a much slower release of sugar and the carbs tend to be full of fiber which helps you feel full for longer. Foods that would fall into this category are things like flax and chia seeds, fibrous veggies like cauliflower and broccoli, along with my favorite thing to bake with, green plantains. The low glycemic index in green plantains makes them the perfect swap for traditional baking flour.

When I first started down the Ketogenic path, a few critics in my life questioned the safety of being in a state of ketosis for any period of time. I had armed myself with the information to be able to have an intelligent conversation with the critics and I even enlightened a few of them.

Just as with any "diet," there are pros and cons. I did my due diligence and spent many hours researching this lifestyle and came to my own conclusion that this was something that could potentially help me not only lose weight, but more importantly, give me my health back.

What works for me, the exact way I do it, might not work for you and it's important to listen to your body and do what works best for you.

I'm sure some of you have done some of your own legwork and are drawing conclusions of your own. I absolutely encourage you to keep learning and continue searching out information.

One word of caution - check your sources.
I personally have a hard time taking information from the mainstream medical community at face value. This is based on my own personal experiences with doctors that were less than competent.

That's not to say all doctors are incompetent. In fact, I urge you to find a doctor who is willing to work with you and is open to alternative treatments. I have found that once I started taking more control and personal responsibility for my health, doctors were more receptive to my suggestions for treatments.

As I mentioned, I am not a medical expert. All I can do is share my own results. Other sources you can turn to include Dr. Jockers, Dr. Mercola and Dr. Axe.

Ketosis

Let me start off with the basics.

The word ketosis may not be completely foreign to you. I remember hearing about it the first time I tried the Atkins Diet in the late '90s. I knew it helped with weight loss but the details of how and why were fuzzy.

I now know that ketosis is a metabolic state that forces the body to rely on fat for its energy needs. People eating a traditional American diet are primarily burning glucose because there tends to be an excess of glucose available to the body. If glucose is available, that's what the body will go for because it metabolizes this the fastest.

Ketosis, on the other hand, forces the body to rely on ketones for fuel versus glucose stores. There is a certain amount of glucose our bodies need for survival, but that does not mean you need to get the glucose from food. Our bodies have been known to survive during long fasts or famines because glucose can be created in the liver from breaking down fat.

Rather than turning to the muscles and breaking them down for fuel, the body will create ketone bodies. This happens when certain hormones cause fat to be released from fat cells in the body where it then proceeds to go to the liver for it to be turned into ketones.

Ketone bodies are the byproduct of this process. The ketone bodies are then distributed throughout the body to places like the brain and other major organs that need glucose to survive. That's why most people do well on a low-carb diet. Pretty cool, right? Our bodies will naturally turn into fat-burning machines.

Who doesn't want to be a fat-burner?

Ketosis vs. Ketoacidosis

Many people I speak with hear the word ketosis and immediately think of ketoacidosis, the dangerous metabolic state that occurs in Type 1 diabetics.
With type 1 diabetes, the body is unable to convert glucose consumed through food into fuel for the body. No matter how many carbs are eaten, the body is starving and turns to the fat to burn. Normally this would be a good thing except the most important hormone needed to regulate fat burning and ketone production is insulin, the thing that Type 1 diabetics don't produce.

Ketoacidosis is the result of uncontrolled amounts of ketones disrupting the entire body. It can cause inflammation, dehydration, and brain swelling. It can be fatal. I have personally witnessed how bad it can be.

My husband has been a Type 1 diabetic since he was 19. When I was pregnant with our son, he went into ketoacidosis and spent five days in the ICU. He had not been taking care of himself and his blood sugar was out of control. There was a point when he was being admitted into the hospital that the doctors told me to call his parents to let them know how bad off he was.

The first few nights were touch and go and my husband was unconscious for most of that time. There I was, 7 months pregnant and watching my husband, praying he would come out of this to meet his unborn son. Good times.

It is possible, however, for a Type 1 diabetic to do well in ketosis so long as he or she has good control over their blood sugar. My husband follows the ketogenic life along with me but does not limit his carbs quite as much as I do. He follows a lower carb diet and has great control over his blood sugar. His blood sugar is more stable now than at any other time in his life because he does not have the huge sugar highs brought on by high-carb meals.

When an otherwise healthy person goes into ketosis, the body becomes an efficient fat burning machine. By limiting carb and sugar intake, the body does what it was intended to do and turns to your fat stores for fuel.

Interestingly enough, going into ketosis can reverse and restore metabolic dysfunction. I have no doubt that I was becoming insulin sensitive and know for a fact that my fasting blood sugar was in the pre-diabetic range for 2 years leading up to my ketogenic life. The very first time I did blood work after the lifestyle change, my levels were well within the normal range. I realized then that there was something significant changing inside of me.

Soon after metabolic issues are addressed, people are less likely to suffer from blood sugar swings and in turn, eat less. Ketosis acts like an appetite suppressant because you're not constantly feeling the need to graze or eat to unconsciously stabilize your sugar levels.

Risks and Drawbacks

People that suffer from an inability to metabolize fat properly shouldn't go into ketosis. Ketosis can be an issue if you are pregnant or trying to get pregnant. Fertility peaks when the body is nourished so ketosis is counterproductive for that.

If you are doing high intensity activities like Crossfit, you burn through your fat stores quickly and then you risk injury as your performance decreases.

Kidney stones can develop if you stay in ketosis for long periods of time. I kicked myself out of ketosis every 3 months in the beginning until I hit my goal weight. Now I cycle in and out of ketosis a few times a month.

Drinking copious amounts of lemon water drastically decreases the risk of kidney stones. This does two things: it flushes the kidneys constantly and boosts vitamin C levels which can also be depleted in a low carb diet.

Making Your Own Decisions

Becoming a fat burner changed everything for me. I'm sure that if I hadn't jumped into the ketogenic diet with both feet, I'd be a confirmed Type 2 diabetic by now.
Knowing kidney stones were possible wasn't concerning for me because of the amount of lemon water I drink on a daily basis (lemon water is a great preventative for stones).

I'm not doing any type of high intensity Crossfit programs and I'm not planning on doing any in the future either. But on the off chance I got the Crossfit bug, I know that I could still do the workouts with the help of a sweet potato every now and then.

Do your own research, listen to your body and decide what's best for you.

The series of events that led me to the ketogenic world are some of the greatest-worst moments in my life. The struggles, the pain, the grief, all of it awful and amazing because it led me right to where I'm supposed to be. There are no accidents.

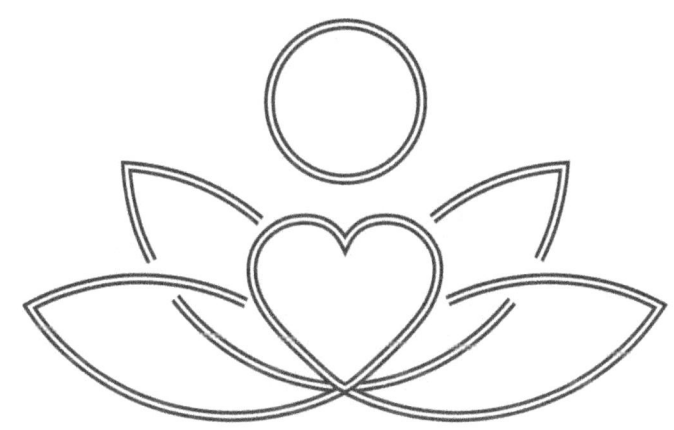

Chapter 3: WHY INTERMITTENT FASTING WAS THE KEY TO MY SUCCESS

Chapter 3: WHY INTERMITTENT FASTING WAS THE KEY TO MY SUCCESS

Not Just What You Eat, When You Eat

Changing what I ate was only the first step. Changing when I ate was another key to unlocking the kingdom of health for me.

When I removed sugars, grains, processed foods and other "frankenfoods", out of my diet, I replaced those things with real foods filled with things like good saturated fats and veggies with nutrients I couldn't get from other food-like substances. I could taste food for the first time.

Then I took things to the next level with intermittent fasting. Everything came alive and in turn, I did as well.

Only the First Step

By making changes to my eating, I started really appreciating food in a whole new way. Food was no longer the enemy. The more I continued to eat this way, the more I appreciated it and lost most (not all) of my cravings for sugary or processed foods. Cake is still my nemesis.

I know my weakness and I become hyper-vigilant whenever I'm around it. Sometimes I cave, but most other times I walk away feeling like a superhero without succumbing to its wicked ways.

Food changes are only one part of the equation.

Conquering what to eat allows you to start trusting yourself to make good choices. Most times, eating out of habit or boredom are ghosts of diets past still haunting your current sphere. Once those ghosts are put to rest, when to eat becomes even more important.

Intermittent Fasting Explained

Intermittent fasting. There. I said it. The f-word of the dieting world. HA! If you said your own choice f-word back at me, I get it.

It wasn't too long ago that I was Camp "6 small meals" and would never have dreamed of fasting, intermittent or otherwise. You may have been taught to eat every 4-5 hours and heard that, "The more you eat, the more you lose."

Well, let me ask you this: how's that workin' for ya?

Everyone freaks out when I say that I do intermittent fasting but I find that I function at a much higher level when I fast for 16-18 hours. There are days when it doesn't happen for a number of reasons. If I'm hungry, I eat. If we have something going on that will be keeping me from being able to break my fast at a reasonable time, I eat. If I make the family plantain pancakes on a Sunday morning, you better know I'm going to eat.

Basically, I stop eating somewhere between 6:30-8:00pm and then I break my fast sometime between 12:00-2:00pm the next day.

Now peel yourself off the ceiling so we can talk about the benefits.

So just what is intermittent fasting? Let me be clear, it is not a diet; it's a way of eating. Instead of eating multiple times throughout the day, you choose a window of time and only eat during that set time.

For example, 16 hours of fasting, 8 hours of eating. During your eating window, you eat plenty of good fats, vegetables, and clean proteins. No calorie counting. You choose quality food to eat.

It may seem like a radical idea but this isn't a new concept. Fasting has been around for thousands of years, often done for religious reasons. I know fasting goes against everything we've been told over the years, but hang onto your hats, cuz your mind just might get blown.

Intermittent fasting has been shown to help with:

- Blood pressure
- Cholesterol, lowering LDL (the bad stuff) and raising HDL (the good stuff)
- Insulin resistance, which can cause metabolic disorders
- Reduced cancer risk
- Boosting immune system
- Increase of fat burning and fat loss
- Weight-loss

One of the biggest health crises of our time, obesity, isn't getting any better with traditional mainstream nutrition advice. With obesity come other metabolic issues like type 2 diabetes, strokes and heart disease. The low-fat, multi-grain, 6 small meals a day thinking is making things worse.

We have children (!) being diagnosed with type 2 diabetes, daily. This used to be a disease for old people. Now, it is a major epidemic with our children, and it's all because of what and when we are eating.

Our bodies are efficient machines and were built to be able to go without food for longer than the 3-4 hours we do now. I'm pretty sure there weren't any 24 hour mini-marts back in the paleolithic era, and humans managed just fine.
The reason is because when we eat, it takes 8-12 hours for our bodies to burn through the glucose it gets from food. Fasting for at least 12 hours overnight allows our body to go from a fed state to a fasted state. In the fed state, our bodies can't burn through our fat stores because we are still digesting food we have eaten that day.

In the fasted state, our bodies are forced to turn to our fat stores for fuel. These fat stores aren't just the love handles around our bellies, but also any fatty deposits near our hearts or livers. These fat deposits are potential troublemakers because the heart and liver were never meant to store fat.

When we continually give our bodies food, it doesn't have a chance to use up the glucose it is getting and in turn, it converts it into fat. It's like saving for a rainy day that never comes.

The good news is the fat we curse can become the fuel we burn. This allows us to lose fat (and size) without sacrificing muscle mass.

Fasting also increases the production of HGH. HGH is human growth hormone, usually peaking in adolescence and dropping as we age. HGH helps us with energy, endurance, and muscle mass. This is why I have more muscle tone now than when I was killing myself in the gym 6 days a week. I was lacking the HGH I needed to get the results I was looking for.

I used to suffer from bouts of hypoglycemia and low blood sugar, but by making changes to my diet, when I did start the intermittent fasting, it wasn't an issue because I wasn't eating things that would spike my insulin. Without insulin spikes, there is no crash or blood sugar drop. Breaking the vicious cycle of spike and crash can be difficult but totally doable. Again, eating the right foods first means this is no longer an issue.

This really just scratches the surface and there is much more to this subject but here is what I want you to know for now: Done properly, intermittent fasting combined with a ketogenic diet will get you the results you've been craving your whole life.

Consult your healthcare professional before trying any of this. And I encourage you to look into the resources I provide at the end of this chapter. Don't be afraid to dig into some of the more scientific medical studies. You will be seeing a lot more information about intermittent fasting being used in conjunction with cancer treatments and degenerative diseases of the brain.

Fasting also allows our bodies to fight off diseased cells. Right now, the FDA is looking to add intermittent fasting to the traditional cancer treatments. When we stop feeding mutated cells, they die off. I suspect this is a major reason I've been so healthy. The old saying "Starve a fever, feed a cold" has merit.

When I feel like I'm getting sick, I make sure to limit what and when I eat, more than I already do. I can usually knock out anything within a day or two. That's a huge accomplishment for somebody that for 45 years would get sick and stay sick. The real point of intermittent fasting is to give your body what it needs, allowing your body to go longer periods without needing to eat.

At no time should you feel like you're starving. If you go without eating even though you are truly hungry, you are at risk for forcing your body into a state of stress.

This is especially important for women because this state of stress is known to cause the production of cortisol. Cortisol has its place in health and is necessary in short bursts to help the body deal with stressful situations, but too much cortisol creates adrenal fatigue and produces belly fat.

Most importantly, fasting is something you can do for the rest of your life. The diet changes are necessary because if you eat junk during your non-fasting times, you might be thin, but you won't be healthy. Our bodies weren't meant to stay in a state of ketosis for longer than 3-6 months at a time. So plan on having a vacation for a week, to break out of ketosis every few months. It will take you a few days to get back in, but that's ok.

Once you reach your goal weight, it becomes even more important to cycle in and out of ketosis weekly. If you've got the fasting thing down, you won't need to worry about gaining weight during those off times. Or if you do, it will only be a pound or two, and it will come right off again, with a few of its friends, when you get back in.

If you are reading this and it is freaking you out, don't worry. You are in good company. Nearly every single one of my clients has resisted me on the intermittent fasting. Everyone has fought me on it. And here's what I say. See for yourself.

Once you start eating well, you will see how it's not really an issue; you do not get as hungry as you used to when you were eating foods that caused your blood sugar to spike. I promise you when you start eating well, you will discover for yourself how it is possible to go for extended periods of time without even thinking about food.

Above all else, please know that I don't, at any time, starve myself. And I don't want you to, either. I eat when I'm hungry. Some days I may go longer than the 16 hours, and other days I won't. I listen to my body and I encourage you to do the same.

Still not convinced? Here are some resources for you:

http://www.mangomannutrition.com/you-are-when-you-eat-intermittent-fasting/

http://www.medicalnewstoday.com/articles/295914.php

http://articles.mercola.com/sites/articles/archive/2014/06/14/intermittent-fasting-longevity.aspx

http://authoritynutrition.com/10-health-benefits-of-intermittent-fasting/

Surprising Realizations

Looking back to my vacations during those first 18 months, it all makes sense to me now. I couldn't understand how I could stray from what I would normally eat and still come home at either the same weight or even down a few pounds. On vacation, I was still fasting. Even if it wasn't my normal full fasting hours, I was still giving my body 12 hours. The 12 hour fast is easy for me just because I usually don't get hungry first thing in the morning anymore.

Changing what we eat is just as important as when we eat. I truly don't believe you can have one without the other. We all have different nutritional needs, but ultimately we all need real food. Eating well and allowing our bodies to do what they were created to do, burn fat stores, will give us lasting results and the health we all want to have to enjoy the rest of our long lives.

Fasting Times

I've done a lot of experimentation to come up with my ideal fasting times. I started with a 12 hour fast, going from 7 or 8 at night, to 7-8 the next morning. I did that for a while before trying to go longer. If I wasn't hungry, I'd push out the time little by little.
As long as I eat well the day before, loading up on fats and veggies, I don't get hungry until much later in the morning.

I do drink plenty during my fasting times, both at night as well as the next day. I have green tea in the morning, along with lemon water and kombucha. I stay away from the kombucha with chia seeds during my fast because chia seeds count as fats. Anything with fat will have your liver working.

When the liver is taking a break, it shuts down glucose production and instead, activates the liver enzymes that help turn calories into heat – hello, fat burner! I don't take my fish oil or coconut oil until after I break my fast, either.

One Day On, One Day Off

There are a few different ways to do intermittent fasting.

Some people do it every other day. On their off days, they eat without worrying about times. On their fasting days, they limit their calorie intake to 400-500 calories. I don't like to worry about calorie counting, which is one of my favorite things about this lifestyle.

I never worry about overeating real foods. For those of you that can't imagine going 16 hours without eating, this may be the perfect way to baby-step yourself into it, especially if you are used to calorie counting.

20-Hour Fast

This type of fasting might work well for those of you who work late. This gives you a 4 hour window in which to eat, preferably one large meal filled with all of the nutrients your body needs. It's designed to match the eating habits of our ancestors. During the 20 hour period, you eat a few servings of veggies, proteins and cold-pressed juices.

I actually like this when I can do it. There are days when I just don't get hungry for whatever reason and those are the days that I'll do 20 hours. I don't do this often because most of the time I do get hungry before then and of course I eat.

During the days when I do make it to 20, I eat enough to compensate for the meals I missed. Again, everyone is different and some of you have crazy schedules during the day and maybe already make dinner your biggest meal so this might be a good option. Others may just faint at the idea of going that long without a morsel of food.

The Next Level

Taking the ketogenic diet to the next level by intermittent fasting helps your body turn into the fat burner it's supposed to be.

Intermittent fasting plays a huge role in regulating hormones as well as reducing your chances of developing insulin resistance (type 2 diabetes), lowering blood pressure, and cholesterol.
The health benefits are numerous and the weight loss is undeniable.

Keep in mind, a lot of the things I do now, I didn't start doing in the beginning. If I had, it might have been intimidating. There are different phases to the process.

If you are a newcomer to the ketogenic lifestyle, give intermittent fasting a try in a way that feels comfortable to you.

Once you've made it through the first month or so, you will see how easy it is to incorporate the fasting into your routine because your body has already started to reset itself.

Your hunger signals will be authentic and trustworthy. Until that happens, it's difficult to even think about fasting. It's something we can address one on one, when the time comes, to figure out the best way for you to start the next phase.

You can schedule a private coaching call with me on my website:

ItStartsWithTheFood.com/work-with-me/

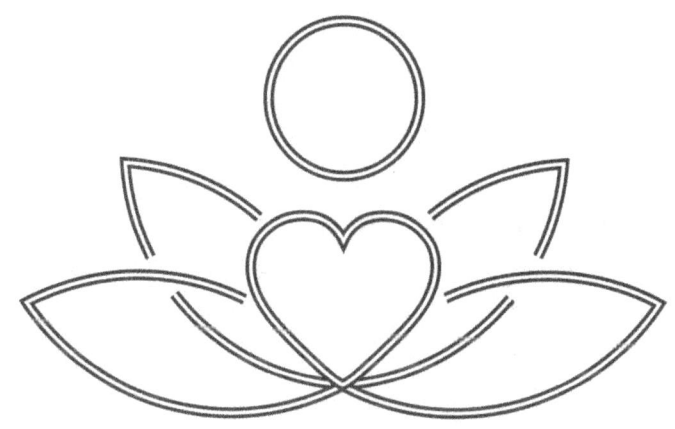

Chapter 4: PREP FOR SUCCESS – SET YOURSELF UP TO WIN

Chapter 4: PREP FOR SUCCESS – SET YOURSELF UP TO WIN

Getting Started

This first week is about laying the foundation for your new life. There are some really important steps to make this transition easier. Some people find detoxing from sugar the hardest part.

When I started the lifestyle change, I was ready.

I'm tough and can be as disciplined as anybody. When I was hitting the gym for 2 hours a day and counted all 1200 calories I was eating, I knew that my lack of results wasn't due to me not trying hard enough.

If you start feeling irritable or sluggish, dig deep and know that it's over in just a few days and you will no longer be a slave to the sugar monster. I chose to feel empowered during those few days: I knew I was finally going to get my life back. Keep that in mind!

You've got this.

So many people have asked me what my secret was, and when I told them what I was doing, they just shook their heads and said they could never do it. It's all about your mindset, though. Give yourself a break and just keep in mind that it's such a short amount of time in comparison to all the time you're going to get from feeling better.

Also - you're NOT alone. I've got you. I'm all in and will be here with info and answers along the way.

How this is Different from Other Diets

Unlike Atkins, I don't eat massive amounts of protein. Too much protein actually converts into carbs!

Your meals should be made up of mostly fats and vegetables with clean proteins. Refer to my It Starts With The Food Recipe Book for more clarity about this section.

For example, a perfect meal would be my Asparagus Cream Soup with Roasted Chicken. The soup is so filling that I don't need to eat that much chicken. You always have the option to add some salad if it doesn't sound like that is enough to fill you up.

Make sure to make your own dressing and use a high quality olive oil. Add some cheese and raw walnuts to the salad and you have a Super Salad. Boil some eggs to have ready in the fridge. Have some cheese, pre-sliced, ready.

If you like sauerkraut or kimchi, make sure you buy some. Fermented foods are great for the body because they help the detoxifying process.

The First Step

Everything starts with you going through your kitchen.

Get rid of the processed foods in your pantry. All processed foods.

My own family does not completely follow my lifestyle, so I do have some organic white rice and organic, gluten-free brown rice pasta on hand for rare occasions. Otherwise, they pretty much eat whatever I cook.

I got rid of anything that would potentially sabotage me. In a particularly shocking move, I got rid of my dark chocolate. I do have a square of raw, live cacao every once in a while, but I have the ability to have a single square and then move on without more. It's got 3 grams of sugar from organic agave per square so I would say that it's probably not a good idea to have it for the first few weeks just to make sure it doesn't trigger the monster.

Sugar is Sugar. Period.

Despite what conventional doctors and food pyramids preach, the sugars in fruit are still sugar and so the body processes it like sugar.

The only fruits I use are lemons (a lot of lemons!), limes, raspberries, and blueberries. I eat the berries very rarely and will only have a handful of them. Raspberries and blueberries have the most bang for their buck, so that makes them the superheroes of the fruit world; they have so many good anti-oxidants and very little sugar, so after the first week or two, you could have a handful in some grass-fed organic yogurt or ricotta cheese with a little vanilla stevia as a treat.

Know yourself and be honest.

Are you somebody that can have just one of something? If not, that could potentially cause problems for you. I also cut drinking waaaaay back. I was drinking 1-2 glasses of red wine 2 times a week. Now, I only drink on special occasions when I'm out. I don't have wine in the house, and I don't miss it nearly as much as I thought I would.

When I do drink, it's usually a vodka tonic (light on the tonic) or red wine and always in moderation.

Before You Start

1. Take measurements

2. Take pictures

3. Track your weight

4. Get a copy of your blood work-ups: You can compare them the next time you get blood drawn

5. Buy some Ketostix, which are test strips that help you figure out if you are in ketosis or not. These are a must. I check my urine every morning when I get up. They are easy and they work. If the strip does not change color, you are not in ketosis; that is a conclusive answer. They are available everywhere. They can usually be found in the pharmacy section by the diabetic supplies or behind the pharmacy counter.

This is a great way for me to stay accountable. Not only does being in a state of ketosis force your body to burn the fat storage but it makes it hard for any disease to thrive.

I was able to stay healthy during the last long, awful winter of illness. When I did get sick, it was quick and mild, unlike before when I would suffer for months at a time.

I can tell you from personal experience that as bad as it might be now, it gets so much better. It's so empowering to see my numbers and know that they are a direct reflection of the work that I put in on myself.

I know that the results of your hard work will motivate you, too.

Your Homework

1. Watch films.

When you have time this week, there are a few documentaries I suggest watching:

- *Fed Up*
- *Genetic Roulette* (free on YouTube)
- *Farmageddon*
- *Food Inc.*

I also suggest checking out DrJockers.com, which is a wealth of good information about the ketogenic life (more on that later in the chapter). These resources will help you fully understand why it's so important to get your body into a state of ketosis and keep it there.

2. Set goals.

I hope everyone has set goals for themselves, whether they are health related or weight related, or both.

It was daunting for me when I first started. I felt like I was putting unrealistic expectations out there for myself, but I had some major work to do. I needed to be audacious and go for broke.

When I was coming close to the end of my first three months, I realized that not only was it likely for me to hit my target, but I was ballsy enough to change my weight-loss goal from 40 to 45 pounds and shorten the time for me to reach my goal. I was originally shooting for the 40 pounds lost by the end of the year and moved the end goal up by two weeks, just in time for my husband's work Christmas party.

When I hit my goal, I felt like I was ten feet tall and bulletproof.

Be audacious and aim for the stars.

Make a Plan

Make a plan for your meals for the first week. This way you won't have to think about it and you will have snacks ready so if you feel like foraging, you have good stuff to grab.

If you haven't yet done this, please get yourself a copy of my It Starts With The Food Recipes book at:

ItStartsWithTheFood.com/resources/.

I have easy meals to make so you don't have to work too hard, and you should make enough to have leftovers for lunch the following day.

Being prepared is the best way to succeed and make the detox process a lot easier. When I went through my first detox, I was not prepared and it was a bit of a struggle. Now, if I go on vacation and have sugar, I know exactly what to do to make the detoxing easy.

What's For Breakfast

For breakfast, if you are a breakfast eater, plan on having eggs with lots of cheese and veggies. If you are not a big fan of eating breakfast, no big deal. Like I mentioned in my section on intermittent fasting, breakfast is NOT the most important meal of the day despite what Kellogg's would like us to think.

Either way, just make sure you are drinking lots of water (or tea, as I discussed earlier).

Lunch Options

For lunch this first week, make it simple.

Some options are egg salad, tuna salad, leftover roasted chicken salad, avocado (I eat this almost every day with cheese, tomato, olive oil, pink salt and apple cider vinegar), or anything else leftover from the night before.

You may want to snack after lunch, so some good options are pumpkin seeds (I like the spicy ones), raw walnuts, raw pecans, pistachios, cut up veggies like cucumbers, celery, any color pepper, broccoli, cauliflower, almond butter or cream cheese, or both, with the celery, sauerkraut or pickles (go easy on regular pickles because they use regular table salt), hard-boiled egg, deviled egg, cheese, and yogurt flavored with a few drops of vanilla stevia (or any other flavor of stevia that you like.)

Dinner IS the Most Important Meal

Dinners are going to be important because they will provide you with leftovers for lunch the following day. This means you may be spending more time making dinner but you will have a few meals out of it.

As I mentioned before, get a good olive oil. It's worth spending a little more for good quality, good tasting oil because you will be using it a lot. There are specialty olive oil stores popping up everywhere and they are worth visiting. I also suggest investing in a yummy balsamic vinegar that can also be used in cooking as well as salads. I use it on my roasted veggies and the kids absolutely love them.

What to Buy

Whenever I refer to dairy, I mean grass-fed and finished, organic, raw (when possible).

When I talk about beef, same thing (except the raw part!)

Chicken and eggs should be pasture-raised and organic. Don't be fooled by cage-free, hormone and antibiotic-free chicken. It's just a loophole that the big food companies use to sell the standard egg or chicken.

I buy organic in most everything, except bananas, plantains, and asparagus. It's a personal choice for everything else. There is a list of produce that doesn't need to be organic, but I choose organic because I'm anti-GMO and until they require labeling, I'd rather be safe than sorry.

Make sure you throw out all of your table salt and replace it with pink Himalayan salt. Even sea salt is now being processed and refined so the only real salt to use is the pink stuff.

Shopping List to Get You Started

A plan! If you fail to plan, plan to fail.

- Almond butter
- Avocado
- BPA-free cup
- Brazil nuts
- Broccoli (raw, cut up)
- Cauliflower (raw, cut up)
- Celery
- Cheese (grass-fed, cut into chunks)
- Coconut flour
- Colored peppers (any)
- Coconut oil
- Cream
- Cucumbers
- Decaffeinated tea (a yummy after-dinner treat)
- Flax crackers (no sugar and all of the carbs are fiber)
- Full-fat yogurt (you can add chia seeds and/or ground flax to it with a flavored stevia and let it sit for 10 minutes for a thick desert) *This needs to be limited to half cup every other day
- Hard boiled eggs/deviled eggs
- Himalayan pink salt
- Heavy whipping cream (to make whipped cream for a "dessert")
- Ketostix (to check your ketones after day 4)
- Kimchi
- Kombucha (a great drink to grab even when you are going through sugar detox. It helps your body detox faster)

- Lots of lemons
- Organic cinnamon
- Organic ginger
- Organic coffee (if you must have it)
- Organic green tea (if you want to replace the coffee)
- Pickles
- Pistachios
- Pumpkin seeds (organic brand)
- Ricotta cheese
- Refrigerator stocked with new foods
- Raw walnuts and/or raw pecans
- Sauerkraut
- Snacks (to have ready to grab)
- Sweet Leaf Stevia (plain and any flavors you might like)
- Water (filtered. Even a Brita-like pitcher will do. No need to get fancy here)

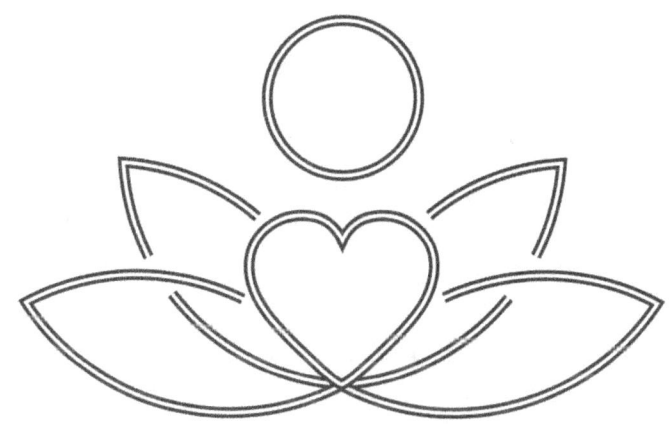

Chapter 5: DETOXIFICATION & THE HEALING CRISIS

Chapter 5: DETOXIFICATION & THE HEALING CRISIS

The First Week

The changes you'll be making once you make the choice to follow the ketogenic lifestyle are more dramatic than you may think.

We all have our own level of attachment to food, on the mental and emotional level, which is enough to cause a struggle and rebellion within during the early days of a detox. Then there are the physical reactions, which sometimes take people by surprise.

When you start out, take things slow. The detoxification brought on by altering your diet in a profound way often causes a healing crisis in the first few days.

Healing Crisis

You may experience some strange symptoms in the beginning. When you start to rid your body of toxins, you may start to feel worse before you start to feel better. This is usually referred to as a healing crisis and is totally normal, so stay the course.

This healing crisis, also known as the "Herxheimer Reaction," is brought about when cells release toxins into the bloodstream and your body isn't able to eliminate them fast enough. The skin, lungs, liver, kidneys, bladder and GI tract get overburdened and in turn this can make you feel like you're coming down with the flu. Symptoms like nausea, headaches, fever, fatigue, and lack of energy aren't uncommon.

Another part of the healing crisis can be caused from what's called a die-off.

This has to do with actual pathogenic organisms like Candida overgrowth (yeast infections), or viruses and bacteria. A die-off can be triggered any time you make significant changes to your diet. Just know that the sicker you are when you begin, the more severe the symptoms from this process will be until the endotoxins are eliminated from the bloodstream.

How Long It Lasts

Just as the severity of symptoms depends on how sick you were when you started, the length of the healing crisis for each person is different.

I've experienced my worst days 2-4 days after I start any detox and it's usually over fairly quickly. Having said that, it can take up to several weeks to get through it completely. If it does take that long, just think about what this says for your state of health prior to starting. Good on ya for averting an imminent health disaster!

People often think the symptoms they're feeling are a sign that something is wrong when, in fact, the exact opposite is true. I say embrace the symptoms in all of their misery. This means you're doing something right!

Detox Symptoms

Now, on to the "lovely" symptoms you may be feeling while detoxing from sugar.

Some of the things you may be experiencing: headaches, foggy brain, lethargy, sweaty, chills, restlessness, irritability, sleeplessness, and overall flu-like symptoms.

It sounds and may feel an awful lot like detoxing from drugs, mainly because sugar is a drug.

Day 3 is usually the worst, but by day 4 or 5, you will be feeling like a champ. You'll get up in the morning with more pep and energy and feel like you've really gone through a transition, which you have.

Things I like to do during any sugar detox:

- Limit any extra activities
- Find a calming decaf tea (mine is chamomile)
- Listen to soothing music (I have a playlist that I go to just for times like these)
- (Probably most important) Let people around me know that I may need some extra TLC and encouragement.

Constipation

Another topic I need to address is constipation. As you make the changes to your diet and you detoxify your body, sometimes it makes things a little ... slower to come out, if you know what I mean.

If you know me, then you know this can be a hot topic because I am not a very happy person if things aren't moving. If you are frequently constipated, then you are in good company. The very first thing I do if I'm feeling backed up is add a warm beverage, usually lemon water, to my meals. Just adding warm liquids helps digestion, and in turn, loosens things up.

Second, I increase my vegetable consumption. The veggies will add bulk and fiber that you aren't getting from the usual suspects: grains and such.

If things aren't moving by day three, add in an organic, caffeine-free, herbal tea designed specifically to get things moving like Smooth Move. They sell it at most grocery stores, whole food stores and online. I drink 1 cup before I go to bed and by mid-morning I'm a happy camper.

Sometimes, I take an over-the-counter chewable tablet that will relieve gas, pressure and bloating that next morning if I'm feeling really bloated and gassy. (Note: if you are unusually bloated and gassy, it may be something in your diet that's not agreeing with you or some inadvertent gluten if you have gluten intolerance).

The fourth thing I add is a stool softener like generic Colace. It is laxative-free but it can definitely help soften things up.

Quick Tips To Fast-Track Your Success

1. Fasting. Revisit chapter 3, on intermittent fasting, if you skipped over it. This is one of my favorite ways to rid my body of toxins and ease any of my detox symptoms. When you fast, all of the energy that would normally go to the digestive system can be used to help your body remove toxins more efficiently.

2. Stay hydrated. I drink a lot of water and I always use lots of fresh-squeezed lemon in it. If I'm in detox mode, I will increase my water intake by 24-36 ounces. Staying hydrated eliminates a lot of the toxins by flushing them out. Make sure your water is filtered.

3. Probiotics. I am a huge fan of probiotics and this is one of the most important additions you can make to your diet. The healthy microorganisms from the probiotics fight the bad bacteria that grow and breeds in your stomach. Cleaning and clearing the gut is the fastest way to get through the healing crisis.

The secret to health, weight-loss and good mental health is getting the gut flora right.

More doctors are realizing that the gut microbiome is actually a second brain to our bodies. It was once thought that serotonin was only produced by the brain. We now know that the gut is responsible for a whopping 90% of the production.

Serotonin regulates mood, gives us a sense of pain, hunger and satiety, as well as gastrointestinal functions. Most of us know that Serotonin is the "feel good" stuff, but how many of us knew that it also helps us with feeling full after eating, keeps things moving, AND helps with our pain levels?

I wonder how many of us are "stress eating" because our serotonin levels are off. It only makes sense that if your gut is out of whack and can't produce the right amounts of serotonin because it's overcome with bad bacteria, pretty much everything else in your body is going to be out of whack as well.

THE KEY TO KEEPING OUR BODIES IN TOP SHAPE IS THROUGH PROBIOTICS.

You can get probiotics through certain foods like fermented foods, kombucha, raw unpasteurized cheese, and kefir. Kefir is like yogurt but has a tangier flavor and more probiotics because of the culturing process. I suggest adding as much of these foods into your diet as possible, but most importantly, invest in a good probiotic supplement.

Over the years, I've also bought quite a few different brands of probiotic supplements and I'm not necessarily stuck on a certain brand as much as the type of probiotics in the supplement.

Be forewarned, if it's cheap, you probably aren't getting what you need. The other thing is you'll want to look for the refrigerated kinds with a minimum of 8 billion/dose as a minimum with 5-10 different strains in it.

Some of the strains you want to look for also have sub-strains. The main strains are Acidophilus, Bifidobacterium and Lactobacillus. I personally have a probiotic with 150 billion/dose and it has 40 different strains in it. I don't think it's necessary for everyone to go out and buy the brand with the most of everything in it... I've just done so much damage to my gut over the years and struggle to keep it in check so I bring out the big guns for prevention.

I can't stress enough how important it is to incorporate a good probiotic into your diet. Hands down, probiotics are the most needed supplement. If you were only going to pick one thing to add to your diet, this would be it.

What would it be worth to you to have health and mental well-being without any nasty side effects? Take the leap and make the investment.

4. Bone Broth. I am such a fan and I always have it on hand. Drinking bone broth will help reduce inflammation; inflammation causes the body to be in a state of dis-ease. You can use vegetable broth if you're a vegetarian, just be sure to use high-quality vegetables. Drink the broth during longer fasting periods. Even though you can buy it, it's best when you make it yourself.

5. Herbs, onions and garlic. herbs, especially bitter ones, like dandelion, parsley, cilantro and ginger are the superheroes of the detoxing world. I use dandelion in my green juice just for that reason. Garlic and onions have anti-microbials full of sulfur which also reduces inflammation caused by the endotoxin die-off. I always put onions and garlic in my bone broth batches and then use even more of them when I use the broth in other dishes.

Why Getting Enough Fat Is Important

Finally, if you are finding yourself hungry between meals, it's probably because you aren't getting enough fat. Fat is KEY for your body to be able to go into fat burning mode and will keep you full between meals.

I suggest adding some cream cheese, avocado, hard cheese, coconut cream, milk, oil, sour cream, yogurt (with flax, chia seeds, stevia and vanilla), almond butter, and regular butter or ghee.

Many years ago, after World War II, some faulty research linked saturated fats to heart disease. In the past few years, it has come to light that this is not the case. In fact, what researchers have found is that people who eat a high-fat, low carb diet, tend to lose weight AND have lower bad cholesterol levels.

There are many ways to access all the right fats without all of the calories.

Here is a list of some of my favorite things to use:

- Avocado
- Beef tallow
- Butter
- Chicken fat
- Ghee
- Macadamia nuts
- Mayonnaise (watch out for added carbs)
- Olive oil
- Coconut oil
- Coconut butter
- Red Palm oil

Make sure to reach out to me if you are having any road blocks.

Visit my website to discover the different ways that we can work together:

ItStartsWithTheFood.com/work-with-me/

Getting Past the Detox

Detoxing is the hardest part of the process but once you get past it, you will start to feel like a brand new person. It may take you longer than others to get through the process.

The length and ease of your detox depends on a few things:

- How much sugar, in the form of carbs or otherwise, you had in your diet before you started. The more sugar you were eating, the longer and more uncomfortable it might be for you to get through this stage.
- How much lemon water you drink. One of the things that will help speed things up is fresh, filtered water with a lot of freshly squeezed organic lemon juice.

THE RULE OF THUMB IS TO TRY TO DRINK HALF YOUR BODY WEIGHT IN OUNCES.

When you are in detox mode, your liver is working overtime to rid your body of toxins so make sure you are helping your liver help you. I use one lemon per day. Every time I fill up my water bottle, I add in some lemon juice.

Trying to find juicy, organic lemons can be a challenge so my suggestion is to stock up when you can find them. I usually buy 7-9 at a time and juice at least 2-3 at a time so I have the juice ready for the next several days.

- Your mindset. I've experienced the healing crisis phenomenon a few different times. Knowing the symptoms and their causes will make it a little easier for you to get through them.

Our bodies are different and what works for me may not work for you. You know your body best. If you listen, it will tell you what it needs.

The reason I recommend that you take measurements and pictures, track your weight and get a copy of your blood work is because the numbers don't lie. And they are the best way for me to track my progress.

You may forget or stray from good eating and bam! Another detox is needed. But at least you have some tricks up your sleeve and will be prepared to do battle.

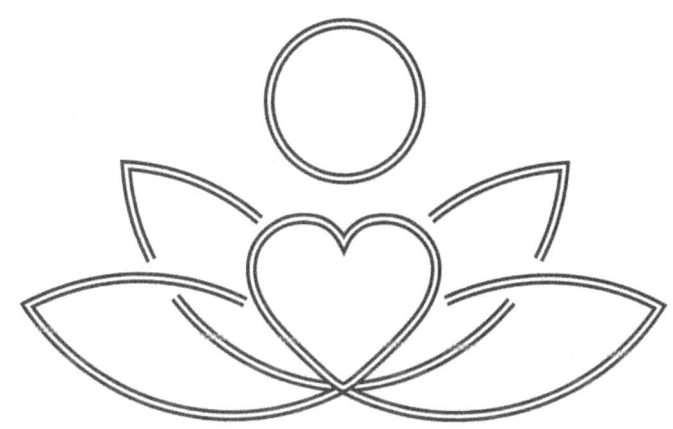

Chapter 6: FOCUS ON FOODS – SOME INCREDIBLE OPTIONS

Chapter 6: FOCUS ON FOODS – SOME INCREDIBLE OPTIONS

Whatcha Eatin?

A lot of days, it's so much more than the food but I always want to remind you how it really does start with what we eat. No amount of meditation or happiness can help the body as much as real food.

I know that most of us are too busy to think about actually taking the time to cook, but if the alternative is ending up in bed or at the doctor because you're sick, what makes the most sense?

I've been averaging an hour per night cooking in the kitchen. It may seem like a lot of time, but I use it efficiently and clean as I go so as not to have a big mess to deal with after dinner. That hour not only feeds 5 people for dinner, but most of the time I get lunch out of it the next day as well.

If I'm making something that either needs to cook on top of the stove or in the oven for any length of time, I will do some prep work for the days ahead. This might be the time to make Plantain Bread if you're making something like Marinara on the stovetop. Or if you're baking something like the Zucchini Lasagna in the oven, make some soup.

Remember that you don't have to eat all of these things as a meal together, but rather as separate meals.

Taking the time to prepare nutritious meals is just half the battle. What foods do you like? What foods are you afraid you will miss so much you might sabotage your entire new ketogenic lifestyle?

In this chapter, I share some of my top foods and suggestions to make eating a little easier... and certainly highly enjoyable... as you make the leap to your new food life.

Broccoli: The Under-Appreciated Vegetable

Broccoli rarely gets the credit it deserves. Most of us think of that bland side-dish restaurants serve lukewarm. But being a part of the cruciferous family makes these miniature trees worth taking a second look at.

I usually end up making broccoli when I'm pressed for time and don't want to think too hard about the veggies. Most of the time, I just shred some grass-fed cheddar onto it, or toss it with some garlic-infused olive oil and feta.

I have also added shredded cheese and ricotta cheese into the mix and it was delish.

Broccoli is one of the best veggies to eat, so don't be afraid to grab some bags of organic frozen broccoli to have on hand for your busy days.

How I Love Thee, Sweet Ricotta

I love ricotta cheese because it's high in the good fats and low in carbs. It's filling and great to eat before the "main course" to ensure you're getting all the nutrients you need.

If you make meat your side and concentrate more on the veggies and give it that extra punch with some good fats, you'll be on your way to having a well-rounded meal.

One more thing about ricotta cheese: I oftentimes eat it instead of yogurt when I want something dessert-like. I use some vanilla stevia with it and sometimes throw in a few raspberries or blueberries. It's not only delicious but yogurt tends to be higher in carbs and too much of it can stall the weight-loss process.

One of my OG's (Original Group) faced a stall and, by going over her food journal, we were able to figure out it was the yogurt that had become her undoing.

Don't get me wrong, I love me some yogurt. But I only eat 4 ounces at a time, loaded up with chia and flax seed, and only have it once in a while.

Just like with most things, moderation is the key.

Did You Say Pizza?

Pizza is one of the hardest things to give up for many people. My fabulous sister-in-law is a creative force in the kitchen. She took my Plantain Bread and did something amazing: She turned it into a pizza!

I've since taken her recipe and added a homemade marinara... I could easily eat this a few times a week.

Like I've said before, having staple recipes makes life easier. It is equally important to add some variety so you don't get bored and start looking to fill the void with some not-so-great options.

The Marinara Sauce can be used in so many of these recipes. Instead of using sauce in a jar (that contains added sugar), this has no sugar and only 2 carbs per serving.

I have used it on top of cheese-baked chicken breasts. I've used it in the Zucchini Lasagna and the Veggie Stack recipe. The sauce is so good that my family puts it on almost everything. My daughter, Terran, said it was so good that she would eat it as a soup.

The beautiful thing about the idea of pizza is that you can put whatever you want on it. If you like veggies, load it up. If you want just sauce and cheese, have at it.

You can find the recipe in my recipe book, *It Starts With The Food: Kickin It In The Kitchen Ketogenic Style* over at ItStartsWithTheFood.com/resources/.

I'd love for you to make it and head over to the Facebook page to let me know what you used for toppings and what you thought of it.

Himalayan Pink Salt

If you have been reluctant to swap out your table salt or even sea salt for Himalayan pink salt, it's time.

I can tell you as someone who has had massive problems with water retention in the past, making the switch changed everything for me.

Once I started using HPS, I was able to come off of my diuretics (medication to reduce water retention). At one point in my life, I was swelling up 10-20 pounds in a matter of days, from salt intake. It was scary and drastic and doctors had no answers so, instead, threw pills at me to take care of the symptoms.

Treating the symptoms but not addressing the cause is a waste of time and money, and takes a huge toll on your body.

It's extremely obvious to me when I'm ingesting anything but HPS because I do swell and retain water. This is one of the reasons I see gains on my scale after eating out or eating foods I'm not personally preparing.

I use the heck out of HPS when I'm cooking and never have issues with swelling or water weight gain.

Other Uses

I had no idea it could be used to reduce stomach acid. When things like heartburn show up, I always look to see if the culprit is inadvertent sugar intake but that doesn't help while you may be in the throes of an attack.

Keep the HPS on hand and heartburn won't be a problem.

Here is a brief summary of the 10 uses:

- Mineral soak. Through the soaking, your body is better able to absorb minerals through your skin that it otherwise might not be able to.
- Soothe away soreness. Through the actual soaking in it, the body is able to use the minerals to help strengthen your bones, skin and tissue that may be contributing to your soreness.
- Detoxification. Again, bathing in it helps draw the toxins out and replace the minerals we are lacking.
- Purify air. Having a salt lamp around you helps take moisture out of the air and acts as an air purifier as the heat from the lamp eradicates potential toxins.
- Irrigate sinuses. Using HPS in a Neti pot helps rid the sinus passages of bacteria that might otherwise be stuck up there (along with the marble from 1st grade).
- Regulate hydration. If you're feeling dehydrated from illness or workouts, grab yourself a mixture of HPS and water and you've got yourself a better sports drink than any currently on the market (without the fluorescent frankenfood colors).
- Lower blood pressure. As long as you're replacing table salt with HPS, you won't have to worry about high blood

pressure. Because table salt is highly refined, it makes it harder for the body to eliminate it. The opposite is true for HPS because it is a naturally occurring mineral.

- Balance pH, reduce acid reflux. I mentioned earlier in the book that lemons are actually alkaline and in turn, can reduce stomach acid. The goal for our bodies is to be in a balanced state of pH and HPS helps with this.
- Improve digestion. HPS can actually increase the body's ability to absorb nutrients in the gastrointestinal tract. The more that happens, the less hungry we are so there's a win.
- Strengthen the body. Just as the soak is important, it's also important to use in food. Just throw out the old white stuff and fully embrace the pink crystals.

Daily Seven

Getting all my veggies in is a daily struggle. Ideally, we should be getting 7 servings of the good stuff and for most of us that seems like a herculean task. I will say that with juicing and adding fermented vegetables in, I'm getting closer… but still probably short 2-3 servings.

I have discovered a few tricks for adding veggies to my daily intake.

Last night I grabbed a big butternut squash, 2 bunches of fresh broccoli, and added that to my pork chops. After roasting the butternut squash with some coconut oil and cinnamon, I added grass-fed butter to the final product and it was amazing.

For the broccoli, after lightly steaming it, I just added some garlic-infused olive oil and salt and I have to say, the fresh stuff is so much better than the frozen variety. My plate was full of vegetables and the pork really did end up being the side dish. Not only did I get 3 servings of my daily intake in just that one meal, but I was full for the rest of the night.

This is probably more like what most of my meals should look like. I had plenty of the good fat with the oils and butter, vegetables were the star of the meal, and the protein was about 20% of the plate.

Usually after dinner, I find myself looking to graze on some nuts or flax crackers... not the case after that meal. I was full, but not stuffed. I was done eating at 7pm and even though I stayed up until midnight, I never got hungry. I had leftovers for the next day so when I break my fast, I will be grabbing some more broccoli, squash, and maybe some flax crackers with cheese. I know that will be more than enough to carry me right through dinner.

Summertime Veggies

I get excited about summer because there are so many beautiful and strange vegetables in season. I love going to my favorite local store to see what they have in stock.

One summer, I was lucky enough to come across some baby eggplants. They were adorable. They were almost too cute to eat! I had never cooked with eggplant and had been reluctant to buy them. Not anymore!

Sometimes, I buy new produce and have no idea what I'll do with them but that's half the fun.

Don't get intimidated by veggies you might not be familiar with. If I see something I haven't made before, I'll Google it while I'm in the store. I like finding new things and introducing them to the family. It keeps things interesting and exciting for me as well as the family.

That's how Brussels sprouts became such a hit in my house. I just sucked it up and bought some one day. You'll never know if you like something until you try it. What's the worst that could happen if you don't like it? You don't need to break the bank when trying new things. Just buy a small amount of whatever it is and then get on your computer and find ways to cook with them.

Soups & Stews

I'm always looking for ways to add soups and stews into my meal planning just so I can use my healing elixir.

I brought out my Chicken Curry Soup recipe last week after multiple rainy days and it did not disappoint.

I also whipped up some guacamole from 2 avocados and we ate that with some flax crackers and it was delicious. I also had some leftover marinara from early in the week that I used for mini-Veggie Stacks. I can tell you, it's another great way to add more vegetables into your day. These little babies can be the main dish, they're that good.

Keeping It Balanced

It's easy to get into a food rut and rely on grab-and-go things like cheese and nuts. I now know the importance of prepping things that are just as easy for me to eat when I don't have the time or energy to do much else.

Having things like soup to throw into a mug, or hard boiled eggs to use in egg, tuna, or chicken salad means I have a few choices and I don't have to think too hard.

If you plan your meals for the week ahead on a day when you have a few free hours, it will go a long way towards your success. If you know what you're having for dinner at least 3 times during the week, you can plan your lunches accordingly.

Doing something as simple as frying up some ground beef with a few seasonings is stupid easy and you can use it in a variety of ways. You can put it on top of romaine lettuce, add guacamole or avocado and raw cheese and voila, you have a taco salad. If want to get a little fancier, you can make some Plantain Bread and add some homemade Marinara (which is really easy to make), sauté mushrooms and top with cheese and fresh basil, and you've got pizza!

There are endless ways to eat it, just pick your favorite. I included these specific recipes in the recipe book for a reason. I know they are easy, good, and keto-friendly.

If you happen to be comfortable in the kitchen, by all means experiment away.

Just make sure the food is part of the ketogenic diet and you'll be fine. If you're in doubt, Google "ketogenic diet" and you will be able to pull up a fairly large list of acceptable food. Remember the whole premise of the ketogenic diet is to keep a ratio of 75% fat, 20% protein and 5% carbs.

I don't think calorie counting is necessary if you're eating a lot of veggies to keep you full but remember that nuts can have a lot of calories in them. So can cheese. There is a fine line between eating the right amount of fat and having food that is calorie dense. Having nuts and cheese are great snacks once in a while but shouldn't be a staple.

If you are eating a decent lunch and dinner, you shouldn't have a need to snack much in between.

You'll be surprised at how easy it is to get fat in. If you have a salad with egg, some raw cheese, avocado and olive oil, you've got the perfect meal. Just make sure to have a few different types of veggies in the salad mix, go light on the tomato and heavier on spinach and romaine, and add some cucumbers.

A fantastic addition to this meal would be a cup of Asparagus Coconut Cream Soup. If you are in need of carbs, add a slice of Plantain Bread covered in grass-fed, raw butter and cinnamon. This meal would help you get the right amount of calories as well as fats, proteins and veggies.

What to Drink

Coffee

If you have to have coffee during the first few weeks, make it count.

Put a teaspoon of cinnamon, some nutmeg, and some grass-fed cream in it. Limit it to 1 reasonably sized cup. I highly recommend cinnamon every morning.

Cinnamon is fantastic for lowering blood glucose levels, boosting metabolism, curbing hunger, it's a natural anti-inflammatory and fights heart disease.

Green Tea

I switched from coffee to green tea. I start my morning with 1 cup of warm lemon water first on an empty stomach because it's a great way to get a little burst of energy. After that, I make my tea. I use 1 organic green tea bag, cinnamon, ginger (powder or fresh), about a tablespoon of lemon, and stevia to sweeten.

Decaf Tea

If you have a decaf tea that you like, I recommend having it at night, after dinner when you might otherwise go for something sweet. Sweeten it lightly with stevia. I have a rooibos pear tea that I absolutely love. It feels like dessert.

Lemon Water

I can't live without my lemon water.

After my morning green tea, for the rest of the day, I drink filtered water and freshly-squeezed lemon. I found a great water bottle that I can take everywhere with me. It's BPA-free, which is very important.

BPA is short for Bispheonl A, which causes structural damage to your brain, increases fat formation, alters the immune system and even causes changes in gender-specific behavior.

My water bottle doesn't sweat and keeps my water cold... even when I leave it in the hot car. I have it with me at all times and fill it up many times throughout the day. It helps curb my appetite, flushes toxins, and alkalizes my body.

Benefits of Lemon Water

Boost to the immune system

Lemon juice is loaded with vitamin C and when your body is in crisis mode and under stress, this is the first thing to go.

If you feel like you may be headed down the virus highway, up your lemon juice intake.

Potassium

Potassium is one of the most crucial minerals our bodies need. Lemons are high in potassium and this helps heart, brain and nerve function. Low levels of potassium have been linked to high blood pressure and heart arrhythmia.

Helps with digestion

Even though it would seem counterintuitive to drink lemon water if you have heartburn, it actually helps with heartburn, gas and bloating. It also helps loosen up toxins in your intestines to promote healthy digestion.

Detoxifies the liver

When you begin to flush out toxins that have built up in the body, enzyme function is boosted and that helps stimulate your liver.

Clear skin

Lemon juice is full of antioxidants which not only keep your skin clear but also helps with eliminating wrinkles.

Lose weight

Between the hydrating effects of the water and the pectin fiber in the lemons, you will find hunger pains diminish or disappear altogether.

Anti-inflammatory

Drinking lemon water helps keep the body in an alkaline state. When the body is in a more acidic state, inflammation happens. Inflammation and disease go hand in hand.

It's an energy drink

Lemons and water work well together to give your body that kickstart it may need any time of day. Try replacing your coffee with warm lemon water first thing in the morning. You'll get the oomph you need without the caffeine crash 3 hours later.

A Word of Warning: Soft Drinks

I have a confession: I was a Diet Coke addict before.

I fooled myself into thinking I had a handle on it because I only had one a day (I should disclose that I do get a cherry flavor Diet Coke on the extremely rare occasion, but I am fully aware of the choice I'm making and I don't go there very often.

Kicking the Diet Coke habit was hard until I found my perfect cup and added the lemon.

Keeping Things Interesting

The key to making this way of eating sustainable for the rest of your life is to keep it interesting.

It's important to have your main, no-brainer meals but it's just as important to expand your horizons and try new things. When you eat real food for any period of time, you'll find that your taste buds change and you will have a whole new appreciation for foods you might have passed on before.

I know there are quite a few veggies I never would have even looked at, let alone bought, in the past. Now, I actively search out new things to add to the list of things I can make at any time.

Please head over to my Facebook page and share the new things you've tried, how you cooked with them, and how it turned out. I would like you to share these new recipes with the group.

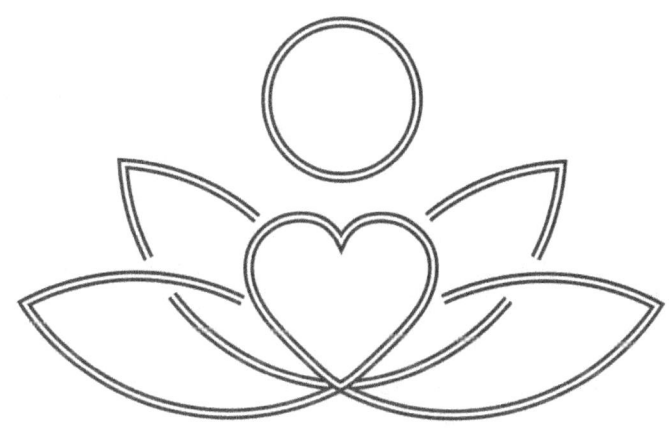

Chapter 7: HEALTHY EATING AND NAVIGATING THE REAL WORLD

Chapter 7: HEALTHY EATING AND NAVIGATING THE REAL WORLD

We all struggle to navigate food in the world outside of our kitchens.

I know none of us want to be "that" person. You know, the one that makes the waiter roll his or her eyes and the whole table groans because the order seems so complicated. I've had to be "that" person over the last 18 months and I admit, it's not comfortable but if I don't look out for myself nobody else will.

There's a great article about how to eat healthy and travel by Dr. Jockers.

Here is the link to his article:

DrJockers.com/how-to-eat-healthy-when-traveling/

This article is well worth a read, and I will discuss my take on many of the points he covers.

A lot of it is common sense; however, it does require thought and planning to really succeed. Think eating beforehand, packing nutritious snacks, and packing digestive enzymes.

The more you travel and eat out, the more you will establish your systems, learn what restaurants have options for you, and, really learn to take charge and feed yourself well... no matter where you are.

What I Eat When Out

One thing Dr. Jockers suggests in that article - that I do not do- is telling your server that you have a food allergy to help ensure you get what you need. I draw the line at telling my waiter I actually have an allergy. I don't want to take away from the seriousness of true allergies. If people start throwing around the word "allergy," I'm afraid that when someone actually does have one, they won't be taken seriously.

While I disagree about the whole allergy thing, I do agree with Dr. Jockers on what to order when out.

I try to opt for wild-caught seafood if it's an option. I almost always order a salad or some other type of veggie and make meat or poultry a last resort or, at the very least, minimize the amount I eat.

I generally stay away from things like soups just because I know how much sodium is used. Often times, things like flour are used to thicken them, so that's just one more reason to steer clear of soups.

As far as salad dressing goes, I've been known to bring my homemade balsamic vinaigrette to restaurants. I might get funny looks, but I know what's in it and can eat it with peace of mind.

I will say I don't do this on a regular basis and most times just go with some type of house vinaigrette. I do drink lemon water like nobody's business so I feel like the two negate each other to some degree. I also don't eat out all that often so I think that helps.

If you are someone who does like to eat out a lot, I would consider bringing your own dressings whenever possible.

Traveling

While traveling, I do as Dr. Jocker suggests. If I'm in the car, I pack snacks for the whole family. I have my own designated go-to snacks, like raw walnuts and cut up cheese.

Whenever we get to our destination, one of the first things I do is hit the local market. I also like the idea of knowing what restaurants are going to be my best options while in the area.

Flying is a little bit more challenging but again, packing snacks for the plane ride will definitely come in handy. You never know when you're going to get stuck on the tarmac or have some other flight delay.

The last thing you're going to want to do is eat the junk they have to offer on the plane.

Any food the airport might have to offer that you can actually eat is sure to cost you almost as much as your airfare. I speak from experience. On our trip to Costa Rica, our flight was delayed by over 2 hours. The whole trip was supposed to be 3 hours and over 5 hours later, I was beyond the point of rational eating. I ate out of desperation and no good can ever come of that.

Plan Ahead

Planning ahead will always be your best option, whether it is for everyday eating or eating on the road. I've said it before, but trying to figure out what to eat when you're already hungry is a set up for food failure. I don't always have a plan per se, but I do know what foods I have on hand to be able to grab when I do get hungry. My trusty avocados are always my back-ups. I also love me some French Brie on Flax crackers.

Those are great choices for me, but everyone will have their own favorites.

I absolutely encourage you to find some favorites and keep those on hand at all times. Keep them simple and easy to grab so you don't have to be hungry AND try to put a plate of something together.

Eating Under Special Circumstances

Whether it's nasty weather, the holidays, time with family or cold and flu season, this chapter will arm you with everything you need to stick to your health goals and ride out any storm - real or imagined.

In Florida, summertime brings daily rain showers and storms that sometimes leave us without power. My clients ask me what they should do food-wise, if a tropical storm, or worse, a hurricane, was to hit. Outside Florida, you may be dealing with other forces of nature, such as tornados or snowstorms.

I'm of the mindset that it never hurts to have some food and water on hand in case you lose power for any length of time for whatever reason.

The items that make the most sense are easy to grab and don't require refrigeration.

That would be manageable if we could eat all of the packaged stuff we used to live on. Now that you have taken on this lifestyle and new way of eating, things get a little trickier.

Here is a list of things that are good to have around in case you are ever looking at a "hunker down" situation:

- Nuts
- Flax Crackers
- Hard Cheese
- Avocado
- Tomato

- Canned Tuna
- Hard-Boiled Eggs
- Veggies, Washed, Cut

My first go-to would be a variety of nuts. Although nuts are high in calories and not something you should be living on, these are special circumstances. No prep needed with these babies.

Flax crackers can be eaten as is, or with almond butter or any other nut butter. Eat flax crackers with hard cheese, like aged Gouda, that doesn't require refrigeration.

Avocados and tomatoes require no refrigeration or cooking. Slice them both up, add Gouda, some olive oil and balsamic vinegar, and you've got one of our staple meals.

If you have a few cans of tuna around, eat the tuna with avocado and that's another meal. Add the flax crackers, and it will almost seem like a fancy picnic.

Let the rest of the family chow down on those chips and cookies while you're enjoying your healthy meal.

If you know in advance that the power is going to be shut off, or when the storm will be hitting your area, hard boiling some eggs beforehand so you can do a quick reach into the fridge without letting too much of the cold out is another option.

A bag of veggies already washed and cut up is another healthy snack option. Again, another quick reach-and-grab into the fridge will help you continue to stay committed to your health goals.

Stress Eating In Emergency or Crisis Situations

If you are a stress eater and being locked up with your family for a few days sounds like the epitome of stress, this would be the time to allow yourself a little treat.

Get yourself a bar of 85% dark, organic, fair-trade, non-GMO chocolate. Chocolate that dark has very little sugar and it is hard to overdo it.

You'll get the benefits of the dopamine without releasing the full fury of the sugar monster. I suggest this because if you are stuck in a house with people eating crap around you and you're feeling like you might snap, this is the better option.

Trust me when I say, those chips you couldn't imagine ever eating again will send out their siren call to you. You see the rocks and yet you go smashing into them anyway. Get the chocolate.

Only a Blip

We obviously can't be prepared for everything. Do your best in any given situation.

Having the staples is a good idea regardless of whether or not we are facing storms or inclement weather of any kind.

No matter what we are faced with, our choices in those moments don't define us. In the big picture, if you do cave and eat some of those evil chips during a raging storm, it will be okay. That holds true for most things in our lives. Whether it be a moment or a day, this is only a blip in your life. It doesn't define you or make you weak.

Do the best you can in any given moment, forgive yourself when you fail, pick yourself back up and start again. And know that I might be hunkering down in some corner of my house, with a tight grip on my sanity and my dark chocolate.

Holidays and Food

Holidays like Memorial Day, the Fourth of July, Thanksgiving, and Christmas… heck, even Easter are synonymous with food, sharing and indulging with family and friends.

I often find myself at food-based functions, and I know the key for me is preparation.

If you are planning on bringing food to an event, make it something that will not only satisfy you, but that others will also enjoy.

My Spinach and Artichoke Dip is one of my favorites. I bring cut up veggies like celery, cucumbers, and colorful bell peppers. I also bring a really good bag of organic tortilla chips for those that want them. This way I know that I'll definitely have something that will fill me up, but is sure to be a hit with everyone else, too.

Plans for Holiday Weekends

I like to cook simple things that make me feel like I have gone out of my way to celebrate whatever the 3-day weekend is for.

A perfect meal for me is to make 2 Roast Chickens with lightly steamed zucchini, red bell pepper and yellow squash (all in season), topped with an olive oil, fresh garlic, fresh dill, lemon and grated Parmesan cheese.

Pancakes for a Sunday brunch. I like to top it with some ricotta cheese and a spoonful of a raspberry jam that I make on Saturday because it is so easy and really satisfies any kind of berry craving you might have.

For those of you that might want something different for brunch, try my recipe for Blueberry Plantain Muffins. These are delicious and really easy to make. It is best when blueberries are in season, because they tend to be juicy and inexpensive.

The most important thing is to enjoy the time with your family and celebrate with healthy food. No need to spend hours in the kitchen!

Eating this way is a lifestyle and something that should not cause you copious amounts of stress when away from the house.

Do your best, make the best possible choices, and then drink your lemon water to undo any damage you may have done while out, on holiday, or hunkered down during a storm.

The essential habit to form is planning ahead, and knowing that the extra time you spend planning and preparing to feed yourself is contributing to your good health and will always be worth it.

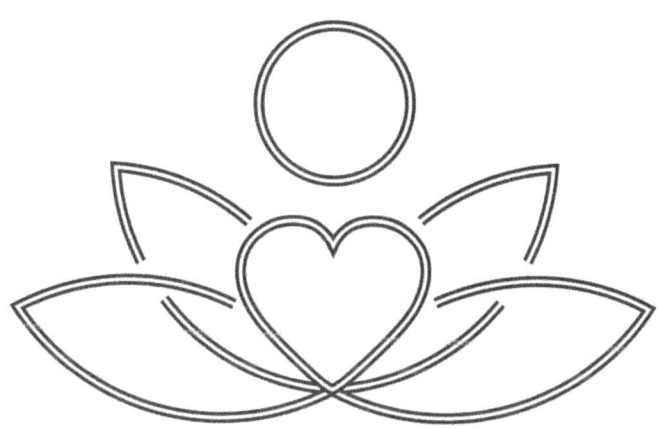

Chapter 8: JUICING

Chapter 8: JUICING

Taking It to the Next Level

I used to have mixed feelings about juicing. My biggest concern was that store-bought juices, even cold-pressed veggie juices, contain too much fruit. Fruit is often used to make the vegetables more palatable.

My concern focused around flooding the body with fruit sugars without the benefit of the fiber to slow down the digestive process. This goes against everything I've learned about keeping the body's insulin levels even and could cause the metabolic disease I've been fighting against with the dietary changes I made.

Despite my best efforts, I sometimes get sick. Not only did I go down last winter, but I took my daughter, Terran, with me.

The one thing I realized during this stress-induced illness was that despite my best efforts, I was still not getting enough vegetables in my diet.

I know how important it is to get my veggies in, I preach it, and I make a concerted effort every day. But I can find it challenging to keep things interesting and switch up my meals because I buy seasonal vegetables.

In the midst of our hazy, snotty delirium, Terran and I were both craving green juice but neither one of us were in any shape to call our local store, place the order, and then get in the car to go pick it up.

As soon as I was vertical again, the very first thing I did was get that juice. I love the mix of spinach, cucumber, lemon, dandelion, and green apple; it's low in sugar and high in nutrients.

As I sat in the parking lot, chugging one of the four bottles I bought, it dawned on me that my body was in desperate need of the vitamins in that green gold.

It was right then and there that I decided it was time to take the plunge into home juicing.

After doing a lot of research, and doing some self-monitoring, I reconciled with my choice. Juicing is the most efficient and effective way to get the nutrients our bodies need without having to eat 8 pounds of spinach or 4 bunches of celery in a day.

Finding the Right Kind of Juicer

I bought a Vitamix a few years ago thinking it would work for a juicer but found that not only did I not like the frothiness of the juice, I learned the high-speed blending actually destroyed some of the delicate nutrients I was aiming to get.

Don't get me wrong, I love my Vitamix but I use it for other things, like mixing my plantain bread ingredients or large batches of soup. If you are in the market for a new juicer, you need to know that a fast-spinning centrifugal juicer isn't as efficient as the slower-moving masticating type. I found that the pulp from the centrifugal juicer was still very wet, and that means there was still a lot of juice to be had from it.

It can be expensive to juice if you aren't getting every drop of liquid out of the produce.

When thinking about making the investment, I had to take a few things into consideration.

At that time, I was spending $5-6 per 12 ounces for my juice. Like I said, green gold. I knew that I could spend $5-6 on produce that would yield at least triple that amount. That would be enough for the entire family for the day. The leftover pulp could be used in a number of different ways, including eating it with some balsamic vinegar and avocado.

After reading many reviews and consulting with people in the know, I bought the juicer which I felt was the best for me, and it cost me less than $200. The machine paid for itself within a few months even if I only juice a few times a week. I thought about all the supplements I can eliminate by adding this to my kitchen counter.

I worry about my growing boys getting everything they need in their food and know that when I'm not looking, the dogs are getting a majority of the good stuff. The boys actually like the green juice and drink it without too much coaxing.

Another bonus.

Not being able to leave the house but craving juice was torture. I will make sure that every person in this house knows how to use the juicer so that will never happen again.

If any of you decide to jump on the juicing bandwagon with me and are local, please share it on the Facebook page.

I encourage you all, as always, to do some of your own research. Juicing may be the thing you need to help take you to the next level in your quest for health and weight.

If, like me, you're having a hard time incorporating enough veggies into your diet, you may want to consider juicing. This is a great addition to our lifestyle for many reasons: It boosts the ability for the body to lose weight, you can drink it during intermittent fasting periods, and it alleviates having to think too hard about getting the greens in.

Juicing is a no-brainer. When you juice your vegetables, you unlock key enzymes that are usually tied up in the fiber and it floods the body with nutrients that would otherwise be hard to get.

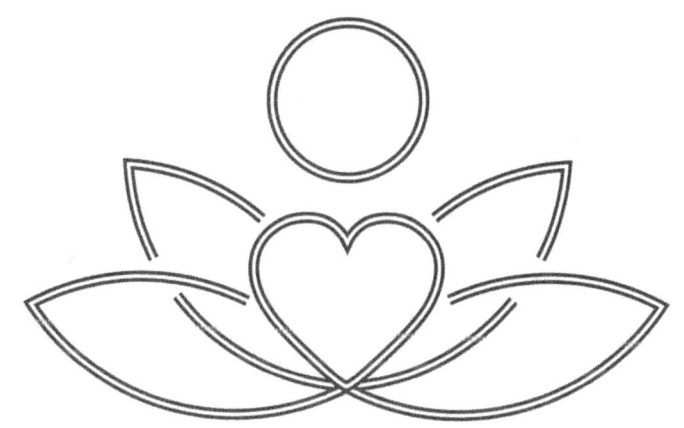

Chapter 9: A NOTE ON EXERCISE

Chapter 9: A NOTE ON EXERCISE

If you are someone who has never liked working out, then you are going to love what I have to say in this chapter!

It is not necessary to exercise for the best results. I didn't and still don't work out. I will do yoga every 3-4 months, maybe.

I see so many people get caught up in working out that they end up missing the most important thing - what they're putting into their bodies. It doesn't matter how hard you work out; if you continue to overlook the quality and type of food you're eating, exercise won't make a difference.

After working out intensely, month after month, 2 hours a day, 6 days a week, and eating what I considered a healthy diet, I didn't lose inches or weight. It was frustrating and defeating. I did enjoy the high I got from the rush of endorphins, but that rush didn't help the disappointment I felt when I got on the scale the following day.

The effort I was putting in didn't match up with the results I was getting. There was a complete disconnect and I had no idea why.

What I've since come to learn is that more isn't always better. In fact, more can be counterproductive and burden the body. By working out as hard as I was, I was putting my body in a state of prolonged stress. This caused my body to produce more cortisol, a hormone produced by the adrenal glands that does serve a purpose when it's really needed.

Unfortunately, most of us are walking around in a constant state of stress and our bodies never return to a relaxed state. By staying in this stress-state, cortisol can cause a myriad of health issues that include high blood pressure, suppressed thyroid function, lowered immunity and... drum roll, please... increased belly fat!

Let me be clear, I'm not a workout hater, I just personally don't enjoy the gym anymore after multiple experiences that left me feeling like a loser (not in the good way).

I do think moving is important though.

The most important aspect of exercising is doing what makes you feel good. If you're working out because you had a piece of cake, stop the madness. You ate the piece, now be at peace with it.

The gym isn't the answer to losing weight. Once you get your diet right, whatever you do to move won't be out of desperation, it will be because it brings you some joy.

Move Your Body

There is a way to help your body without putting undo stress on it. For me, yoga turned out to be one of these ways. It is an unlikely favorite form of movement for me. I say that because I'm really uncoordinated and was horrified at the thought of attempting some of the poses in a class, with actual people around to see me.

What helped me get over the fear of humiliation was a beginner's yoga DVD, gifted to me at a time when my health was really poor and it helped ease me into the world of Downward Dog and Warrior Pose.

Part of the health crisis I was experiencing was a rapid heartbeat and high blood pressure swings. Through this type of movement, both of those things settled down. I also had my first real taste of meditation.

Yoga and meditation go hand in hand. When I was trying to hold a pose, not fall over or collapse onto the floor, I found I needed to get out of my head and become fully present in the moment and focus on my breath. This is meditation.

Swimming

Another of my favorite things to do for movement is swimming. I've had a love for the water as far back as I can remember. There's something incredibly soothing and relaxing for me as I glide through the water with a playlist created just for swimming, playing in the background.

This also did wonders for my blood pressure and heart rate. Even though I would get my heart rate up, it didn't bother me because it was supposed to be higher from exercise. The elevated heart rate was an appropriate response to the movement I was doing. What bothered me was having the heartbeat of someone going to town on an elliptical trainer while I was trying to sleep.

Instead of focusing on things like cardio, go for interval training. You'll be able to knock out an effective workout in 20 minutes or less. A perfect example of this is swimming at full speed for one minute and then returning to a slower pace for the following 3 minutes. Continue to do this for 20 minutes.

Our bodies were built for this. And it provides the same benefits you would get from a traditional cardio workout without putting your body into a high-stress state for prolonged periods of time.

I choose to move in ways that make me feel good without worrying about what it's doing for my waistline.

Do what you love just because you love to do it and you can't go wrong!

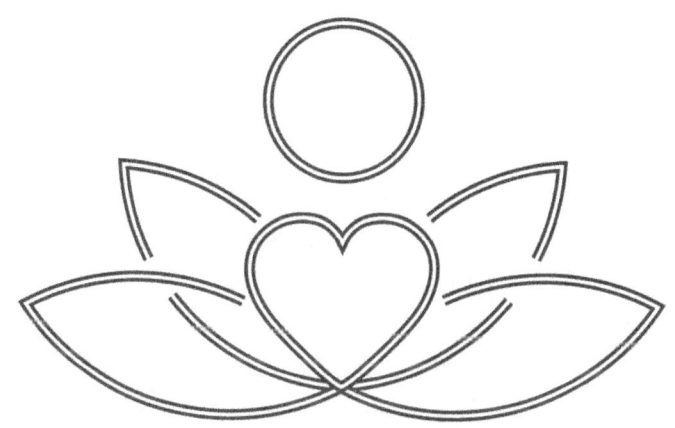

Chapter 10: BEYOND THE FOOD – FINDING OTHER LIFESTYLE CHANGES

Chapter 10: BEYOND THE FOOD – FINDING OTHER LIFESTYLE CHANGES

Mindset

If You are Struggling/Your Monkey

Oftentimes, clients will come to me when they are struggling. The one thing that sticks out to me after having these conversations is that there may be some monkeys on their backs that they can't shake… and those are the things keeping them from progressing.

When I refer to your "monkey," I'm talking about the thing that you struggle with. It might be a sweet coffee drink, cake or potato chips. Everyone has a monkey, you just need to figure out yours.

When I started, my monkeys were coffee and icing. After having some time to reflect, I realize there were more than just those 2 things. I really loved having one Diet Coke per day. I also craved things like ice cream and peanut butter. I had several monkeys but some were harder to shake than others.

I wanted to change more than I wanted to cave into the cravings. I read all of the information out there and implemented the changes because I knew how important each of the little things were to the overall picture.

I still allow for a few of these things every once in a great while, but there are certain things that are non-negotiable, like peanut butter. Peanuts are in the legume category. Legumes contain phytic acid which causes issues with absorbing nutrients. Peanuts are also highly susceptible to contaminants and a mold, Aflatoxin, a known carcinogen linked to liver cancer.

Icing and ice cream are a once-every-6-months type of thing. I'll enjoy a cup of coffee once a month and Diet Coke isn't even on my radar. There was a time when I told you all that if I went to my favorite burger joint, I was most definitely getting a Diet Cherry Coke. But even that has dissipated over the years. A big part of the reason is because when I was getting it, I would pay almost $3 and only end up drinking 1/3rd of it anyway - literally hard to swallow on both accounts.

Recognition to Start

By recognizing what you want and need to make a lifestyle change, you have begun loving yourself.

Changing what you eat is just the beginning. As you start to become fully present in your life, aware of everything you put into your mouth and body, other changes will become easier.

You will recognize stressful situations and people for what they are and you'll feel your body react. You will be so in tune with yourself, you'll be able to feel your blood pressure go up as your adrenaline spikes, like it's supposed to when you're in a fight or flight situation.

Those adrenaline spikes create cortisol and cortisol is converted into belly fat. That belly fat is a silent killer. Isn't that enough to make you rethink the things in your life not bringing you joy?

And remember, sometimes the situation isn't necessarily "bad," you might just need to find the joy in it. For me, my boys can get me wild and definitely send me to Crazytown. During these times, I need to get centered and get right in my head and remember they are my loves. They may not be bringing me joy while they refuse to get out of bed after I have been screaming at them for 30 minutes, but when I see them happy and hear them laughing and they hug me "just because," that's where my joy lives.

It's a process and I'm so not perfect at it.

Add Joy While Subtracting Pounds

What is it that you're doing to add to your life?

Have you been meaning to add meditation into your routine, but still can't manage to fit it in? Are you journaling when you're frustrated or are you stress-eating? Have you been celebrating your successes or comparing yours to others and falling short?

One article that really resonated for me is called "6 Universal Principles That Will Set You Free" that I found on TheSpiritScience.net.

Here is their list of 6 things:

- Action. "Take action towards those things that fill you with excitement and enjoy. Joy attracts joy. Flow attracts flow. Taking action leads you to action in new and related areas of life."
- You attract more of what you focus on. This is all about the law of attraction. Are you focused on what you want or what you don't want?
- Taking responsibility. "This principle of taking responsibility bears fruit in any situation. It stops bad situations from creating animosity and disrespect. It turns a bad situation into a situation of respect and growth. It becomes a situation that fulfills the 4th need of Maslow's pyramid – Esteem."
- Acceptance. When you learn to go with the flow, life is easier all the way around. The more you fight something, the harder it becomes. It's the whole "swimming up river" thing.
- Integration. If you can get away from judging situations as good or bad, you can start to see and appreciate all sides. This becomes your humanity that will serve you in your happiness through this experience we call life.
- Coming back to baseline. This ultimately means having and achieving balance. It's important to be in a state of action but it's just as important to slow down to see where all of that action has led you. Quieting the mind, enjoying the view, rebooting the soul for the next marathon ahead.

I will leave you with this:

"As human beings, our greatness lies not so much in being able to remake the world…as in being able to remake ourselves." ~ Mahatma Gandhi

Meditation

When I started making all of the food changes in my life, I realized there was so much more to me than just the physical body.

Looking good was obviously one of the biggest driving forces for me to make changes, but I could feel something bigger happening inside of me and I knew I needed to nourish it. I suspect when I began to feed my body real food, it woke up and screamed "I'm in here-feed me, see me, heal me!" I began searching for ways to fulfill that command.

Then I found meditation. Meditation helps to center me and reminds me I have more power than I may feel in any situation. The power I have is how I let things affect me.

I've heard from many of my clients about life situations they have had to deal with and I can totally relate. I want you to know that I see you, I hear you and you matter.

Life is a series of events, some good, some tragic, but it makes us who we are. Each situation gives us an opportunity to remake ourselves. We don't need to be defined by our failures or tragedies. Just as our successes don't define us either.

These lifestyle changes I talk about are so much more than just food.

When we start caring enough about ourselves to change what we eat, it's only the beginning. I know for me food was the launching pad for unimaginable happiness and joy. I started caring enough about myself to distance myself from things and people that didn't fit in my life anymore. I like to say, "If it brings you joy, do it, if not, walk away."

Where to Start

Meditation comes in many forms. In the simplest terms, it is a matter of being able to quiet the day-to-day noise that acts as a distraction from our higher selves.

I know when I'm listening to my inner voice, I tend to be happier and more at peace with situations out of my control. I remember to breathe deeply and take a minute to respond instead of reacting immediately.

You might ask yourself, "What does this have to do with health and weight?" All I can tell you is that I strongly believe lifestyle changes must be a mind, body, spirit combination. I don't think you can have lifelong changes without addressing all of those connections.

How many people do you know that are healthy or skinny, or even both, but still lack happiness and peace?

Prayer is a form of meditation. Standing in the shower, quietly, letting your mind go and allowing your inner voice to speak, is meditation. There is also the more traditional guided meditation. All of these are great as long as you are practicing them daily.

Benefits of Meditation

On a physical level, meditation:

- Lowers high blood pressure
- Lowers the levels of blood lactate, reducing anxiety attacks
- Decreases any tension-related pain, such as tension headaches, ulcers, insomnia, muscle and joint problems
- Increases serotonin production that improves mood and behavior
- Improves the immune system
- Increases the energy level, as you gain an inner source of energy

On a mental level:

- Meditation brings the brainwave pattern into an Alpha state that promotes healing. The mind becomes fresh, delicate and beautiful.
- Anxiety decreases
- Emotional stability improves
- Creativity increases
- Happiness increases
- Intuition develops
- Gain clarity and peace of mind

- Problems become smaller
- Meditation sharpens the mind by gaining focus and expands through relaxation
- A sharp mind without expansion causes tension, anger and frustration
- An expanded consciousness without sharpness can lead to lack of action/progress
- The balance of a sharp mind and an expanded consciousness brings perfection
- Meditation makes you aware that your inner attitude determines your happiness.

Guided Meditation

Finding a guided meditation is also a useful tip for anyone new to meditation.

Deepak Chopra and Oprah Winfrey frequently host 21-day meditation courses online, and several other teachers like Louise Hay, Doreen Virtue, the late Wayne Dyer, among others, have guided meditations available for free online of if you subscribe to their podcast.

But I Don't Have Time…

The guided meditations are 15-20 minutes long. You can do them anytime during the day and you can even download it to your phone. You've already committed to big lifestyle changes, what is 20 minutes per day, really, in the grand scheme of things?

What if spending this small window of time during your hectic day helps you get back to a place of joy and happiness? Isn't it at least worth trying?

Make Time for Yourself

Recently, I booked a trip with a group of women that I've wanted to take since 2014, when my sister and friend went on this same retreat. All these women were looking to work on themselves, grow and evolve through the guidance of an amazing leader.

I felt guilty and selfish for even thinking about going on this trip because it was a costly investment. I procrastinated about it too long and eventually all of the spots were taken.

I was kicking myself for hesitating. I deserved to make choices that reinforce my growth, my belief in self and my wellbeing.

What had me pause was the money and the potential for my husband to resent my time away from him… and then I realized I would never think twice about spending the money on my family, nor would I begrudge my other half for wanting to work on himself, away from the family.

Two months after the deadline to register, the woman leading the group posted on Facebook that someone had cancelled, leaving one spot open. I saw this as my sign and after talking to my understanding husband, I booked it. As soon as I made the decision, I felt this wave of peace and joy. I knew at a cellular level that this was exactly what I needed. Not only would it fill me up with knowledge to be able to share with my clients, but it would give me time to focus my energy on personal growth.

I know it isn't always possible to plan trips and attend expensive excursions, retreats, seminars or events but I can tell you, having something to look forward to - even if it's just time at the house when nobody else is around - can go a long way to getting you through uncomfortable moments.

Make time for yourself. Sometimes feelings of unease come up because you aren't paying attention to fulfilling your own needs first and foremost. When that happens, it's hard to be anything for anybody else and this can leave you feeling empty and drained.

My biggest takeaway from the retreat was the importance of connection and community.

I've done life alone for many years. My husband and my sister have served as my tribe for the past 20 years and I couldn't be more grateful to have them in my corner. But, when I was standing in a circle with 40 heart-centered women, with no agenda, just love, I felt a peace I didn't even know I was missing. My spirit came alive with remembering how connected we all are.

A lot of us spend a majority of time focusing our energy on what makes us different from one other, completely overlooking the similarities. I say to you, go do the scary, selfish, hard things. You never know when you'll have the awakening and find your tribe.

Sharing Your Life

There are times in my life when it feels like the Universe is dominating my energy and not in a good way. My life is full of amazing things, people, and opportunities. Sometimes there doesn't seem to be anything to point at and say, "Ah, there it is. This is what's keeping me in a funk."

However, I do know one thing for sure... this moment is important and I need to pay attention. If nothing else, this helps me on my path to empathy and understanding when others are suffering too. How can I possibly be of service to others if I never experience the lows along with the highs?

I want you to know that you are NOT alone.

I was telling a friend that sometimes we all get funky together and those are the times we should be looking to each other for support. Yes, misery loves company, but shared experiences create bonds that make life a little easier to manage.

As we face life's hurdles together, we grow together. Make sure you include regular contact with friends and communities to help you solidify the changes you're making. And, speaking of...

Reinforcements

My job is to constantly look for new ways to improve all aspects of our lives.

I believe that when you conquer one part of your life, it tends to reveal other parts that need work. Maybe some of the funk has to do with realizing that food and weight aren't the end all, be all. Kind of like the game Whack-a-Mole, one more thing pops up and we need to confront it head on.

I've been known to revert to the old thinking, "Maybe if I'm really quiet, it will go away." It never fails to backfire because it ends up being the thing that keeps me up until all hours of the night. I will tell you that the world seems insurmountable when I haven't been getting enough sleep.

I also know lack of sleep causes weight gain and takes a toll on the immune system.

I'm sending reinforcements out to you in case you ever feel like this.

I came across a fabulous article from Wake Up World that might come in handy on those dark days:

"8 Emotional Patterns That Can Disturb Our Inner Peace"

It's all about emotional patterns that can disturb our inner peace. Whenever you get into a funk, this may be just the thing to help you figure out what it is keeping you from experiencing full joy in your life. I know it helped me channel some of my crazy, all-over-the-place thinking and gave me the tools I needed to do some introspection. Sometimes, all it takes is just sharing how you're feeling without fear of being judged.

Putting it out there means you are casting light on some of the darkness and the shadows shrink.

I'm sending love and light to you all in hopes it allows you to illuminate any lingering darkness. One more thing to remember is the old saying, "What a difference a day makes."

Today doesn't dictate your tomorrow or define your yesterday. A change in attitude and perspective goes a long way on your journey.

Helping You Have it All

Today is all about you.

What have you been doing recently to add to your spiritual, physical, and emotional well-being?

Are you celebrating the little successes you're having or are you berating yourself for not being as successful as someone else?

If we constantly look outside of ourselves for validation, it becomes easy to focus on our setbacks instead of celebrating our own moments of personal success.

Object-referral is the term used for seeking validation from an outside source. The only validation we should seek is from the voice of our highest self. Your opinion about yourself is the only one that really matters. How many times has someone told you how great you look and yet you still felt ugly?

Exactly.

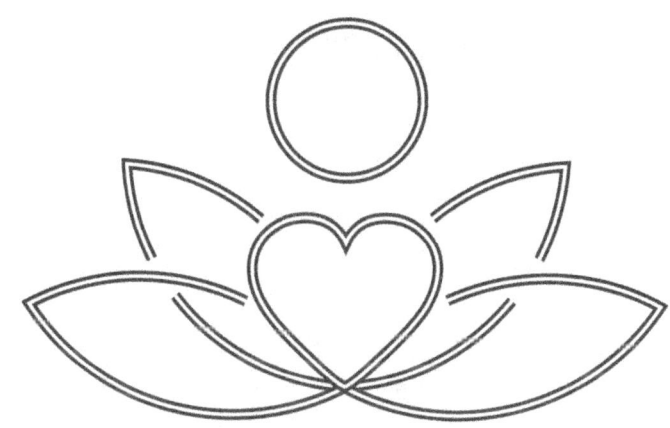

Chapter 11: IT'S ONE THING TO MAKE CHANGES…IT'S QUITE ANOTHER TO GET RESULTS

Chapter 11: IT'S ONE THING TO MAKE CHANGES...IT'S QUITE ANOTHER TO GET RESULTS

Now it's time to address the results, or lack thereof, you may be experiencing.

The other day, a fellow Ketogenician told me she wasn't having consistent losses. I asked her how closely she was sticking to the lifestyle and she said 95% of the time. I said she would then see 95% of the results.

I was wrong.

After talking it over with another friend, I realized that when you are only sticking to it for 95% of the time, you really only get about 70% of the results. One day or one meal means you're putting your body in a place where it then needs to reset itself. That usually takes 2-5 days. So, if you have a specific weight loss goal with a time frame in mind, remember that 5 minute cheat may set you back 5 days.

Before indulging, ask yourself, "Is it worth it?"

This is a marathon, not a sprint. These are habits you are trying to establish for a life of healthy eating. There will be plenty of time in your future to indulge every now and then. Doing it, especially while you're trying to reach goals you've set for yourself, may not be worth the few minutes or few bites of a "treat."

When I started these changes, I knew I was going to indulge, in moderation, when I went to Mexico in October. That means from May until then, I was very strict about my food choices. In turn, I got the results I wanted, and then some.

By that time, my body was also becoming a true fat burner so when I did eat a few things I normally abstain from I didn't gain more than 2 pounds during my 8 nights in Mexico. I stayed in ketosis for more than half the time I was there and then was able to get back into ketosis within 3 days of my return.

Keep the bigger picture in your head at all times so when you're faced with temptation, you might find it easier to turn it down without feeling sad or depressed because you "can't" have it.

It's a choice.

Getting to Know Your Body

You know better than anybody what works for you and what doesn't. It's just a matter of paying attention to the cues and adjusting your diet accordingly.

A food journal is great to keep you honest and accountable. It should include EVERYTHING. Every time something goes in your mouth, write it down. Water, kombucha (and be careful that you aren't getting more than 4 grams of sugar per serving in a day from it), coffee, tea, etc., are all things to put in the diary.

It's easy to have seemingly harmless things in our diet be the saboteurs. The only way to know if it really is harmless is to keep track and use your tools.

Most importantly, food should be fuel for your body. It is the most important part of your life and should be prioritized as such. Having a well-rounded diet will keep you from becoming deficient in any one thing.

If you want to continue to see improvements in your health and weight, you don't have the luxury of being a picky eater.

You are Unique

There are many things that benefit us all, like eating organic, real foods and drinking lots of water.

Other things are more individualized like coffee and carb intake. Oftentimes, there can be hidden booby traps, like coffee, that can keep us from breaking through weight loss stalls.

This isn't to say that everyone needs to give up their cup of organic coffee (and I do mean organic and cup), but if you've adjusted everything else in your life first, this would be on the "naughty" list.

I know a few of you might be thinking about throwing in the towel at just the thought of giving up your beloved coffee, but remember, there are quite a few things that we need to look at before going to that dark place.

Just as ketone sticks are tools, so are things like scales and measuring tapes. Sometimes the scale might not show a big loss for the week, but you notice that you, all of a sudden, have more room in your clothes. I suggest taking out that tape measure during those times. It serves as positive reinforcement and helps you to stay committed to the new lifestyle.

The ketone strips are great if you are adding in new things like flax crackers or wanting to have some sweet potato every now and then. I always like to monitor weight and ketones when adding in new food so I can see exactly how much of something I can actually eat without it throwing me out of ketosis or causing weight gain.

In the case of my brie, it took a few months of eating it... a lot... before showing up as a trend of weight gain on the scale. At that point, I knew it was time to slow our relationship down and only see each other on occasion.

My heart still hurts.

Better Days

My life has been a series of moments and events that I used to classify as "good" or "bad."

Now, I know those are limited labels for lessons I that I had yet to realize. I've gotten to a place where I know for certain there is a gift every time I'm faced with challenges, even when I can't possibly imagine what that gift might be. Usually, the harder life hits me, the greater the gift.

This was the absolute truth for me when I changed the course of my life by getting my weight and health under control. I've realized what I do during those difficult times doesn't define me. Sometimes I rise to the occasion and handle my business like a boss. Other times, I fall short.

When I fall short, it's usually because my priorities aren't in order.

My hope for you is that no matter what you're going through, you know there are better days on the horizon.

It can be easy to throw in the towel when life gets rough. Those thoughts have crossed my mind on more than one occasion. But the pain of how things used to be serves as the catalyst for me to continue on my journey.

Whatever you did or didn't do yesterday shouldn't keep you from making better choices today. Each day is a new chance to get it right. Whatever it is that you're trying to get right, I hope yesterday doesn't jade the way you look at this new day and new opportunity.

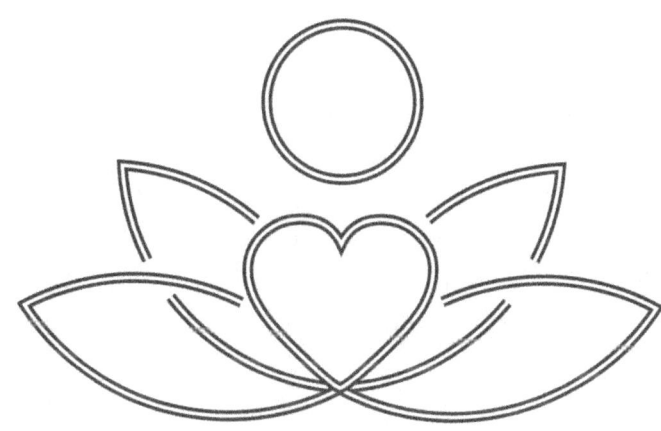

Chapter 12: MAKING IT STICK

Chapter 12: MAKING IT STICK

I find that whenever I try to implement new things into my life, no matter what it is, I need to have the discipline of a monk… especially in those first few weeks… in order for the changes to stick.

I'm reminded of this every time I add in something new to my routine. Recently, I started a 21-day yoga challenge and by day 3, I found myself too busy to do the 15 minute routine. Seriously?!

Day 4 was a different story because I really wanted to make this a permanent part of my daily routine. So even though it was 11pm before I found time, I did it. The payoff was immediate. I felt my whole body loosen up and my spirit lighten. Part of it was the actual yoga, but an even bigger part of it was because I had follow-through.

Just wanting something isn't enough to manifest it. Change and growth require a constant state of doing instead of wanting.

Easier Said than Done

I'm not naïve enough to think that this is easy for you. Nothing worth doing rarely is.

Speaking my truth and then following through with it is challenging for me. I'm inherently a people pleaser, or at least I was for most of my life. So for me to set boundaries and then stick to them when I could be disappointing people… this is my definition of uncomfortable.

What I know to be true is that every time I find myself in a situation that is not in line with how I see my life now, I feel like I'm spending a little piece of my heart and soul. I love myself enough now to know these sacrifices are a betrayal to my spirit.

I wake most mornings (not all, for sure) with the intention of spreading joy and in return, receiving joy. This feeds my spirit and elevates me to even greater heights of happiness.

For me, there is nothing more fulfilling than having a symbiotic relationship with others I come in contact with. Symbiotic is the key word here.

I know you all have encountered people I like to call "Energy Vampires." These are people that no matter what you do, you find yourself spent and exhausted by just spending time around them. None of us want to be that person, but more importantly, we need to recognize these people for who they are, and love ourselves enough to let them go with love.

A relationship with anyone or anything should leave us feeling better for being a part of it. The give and take is what allows us to give without feeling empty after it's over.

It's the Little Things

If you're anything like me, it's easy to get gung-ho in the beginning of things; the excitement of the changes to come is enough to get me motivated. Sometimes, that motivation is enough to carry me through that crucial 2 month period to develop it into a habit. And sometimes, that motivation doesn't help at all.

Yep, 2 months, not 21 days like we were all led to believe. 8 weeks versus 3 weeks is a huge leap. What this means is that if there is something you want to add or change in your life, you'll really need to give it all you've got for 60 days. During those 60 days, you'll develop a habit that will hopefully carry you through periods in your life when you may not be as vigilant as you should be.

When you hit a bump and get off track, that habit you developed will help you get back on board without losing too much momentum.

While you're still caught up in the newness bliss, that's the time to make a new routine that's manageable.

If you're in Phase 1 of making dietary changes, figure out what days you'll have time for grocery shopping and stick to it. Have another day (or maybe the same day as shopping) that you'll do some meal prepping. Set aside a few hours each week to just do some cooking.

I normally have my time scheduled fairly well, but when I found myself with a few extra hours (how did that happen?) one Monday, I made Plantain Bread, Asparagus Soup, Roasted Butternut Squash, and 2 packs of Easy Chicken Thighs.

It only took 2 hours to make all of that food, enough for dinner that night and meals-at-the-ready for the next few days. This bonus cook-off meant I had time to spend my entire Tuesday working on putting my cookbook together.

It's the little things, like having a schedule, which will help you recreate the life you want.

Back to Basics

I'm not immune to straying away from the things that brought me so much success. It usually happens when I find new things to introduce to my diet or I start relying on too much of one thing, like brie.

Brie has officially become my new arch nemesis. I have virtually no self-control when I eat it. I can polish off half of a wedge in one sitting. It's high in fat, calories, and sodium. It's a trifecta… and not the good kind.

I didn't realize it was causing problems until I looked down at the scale and saw a steady increase and not my usual fluctuations.

The good news is because of the routine of weighing myself EVERY morning (unless on vacation) I was able to see the trend and address it. Anytime you feel yourself slipping from everything you've built, just go back to the basics and begin again.

Taking Inventory

In all of my years, I have recreated my life more times than I can count. Each time I did, it required me to take an honest inventory of my current situation and reevaluate my priorities.

I had to ask myself if I was doing everything I needed to in order to grow in the direction I wanted or was I being complacent and expecting things to just happen? Was I willing to let go of old habits, get uncomfortable, and bring Heather 2.0 into being?

We all have things in our life that we want to change and I feel like that's a good thing. Being comfortable leads to stagnancy and I firmly believe we were meant to be creatures of movement and action.

Now is the time to take your own inventory. What are the things in your life that no longer fit the vision of the person you aspire to be? Are you taking action or sitting on the sidelines, crossing your fingers in hopes that your dreams will come true? Make a plan, and then make it happen.

Taking Action

A great way to work on the mind, body, and spirit, is by taking action. Action can come in the form of meditation, journaling, physical movement, seizing opportunities as they present themselves, or even just reflecting on your journey to this point.

Instead of looking around you to see where you're at compared to everyone else, take that time to see where you're at compared to where you were.

If the scale isn't reflecting what you think it should, grab the measuring tape and take measurements. If you didn't take measurements in the beginning (tsk, tsk) then grab that pair of shorts or pants - the ones gathering dust in the furthest corner of your closet - and see how close you get to buttoning them. I remember trying on different sizes in my closet as I lost weight and had a few pairs of shorts that, almost in slow-motion, the button finally reached the button-hole.

The journey to get there was part of the fun. I never knew what day it was going to be when it finally happened and when it did, the sense of victory was one that nobody could've given me. This was all mine.

Slow and Steady

I want to reiterate that I, personally, never had big drops but steadily lost 1-2 pounds per week. So no matter which category you fall into, it's all about personal successes.

It's hard not to compare yourself to others, but it's kind of like driving next to the speed racer who weaves in and out of traffic, only to end up at the same stop light together. If you experience a few big drops, prepare yourself for leveling out to average 1-2 pounds per week. Ideally, you should all be aiming for that goal.

It's been shown when you have that average you are more likely to keep the weight off. Having said that, you should be able to keep the weight off just because this is a lifestyle change, not a temporary fix.

Information Overload

The information in this book is important to reference and re-read. There may be a lot of things that didn't make sense the first time you read it but now, after being in the lifestyle for some time, the light bulb might come on.

You are all busy - me too - but I don't think it's unrealistic to set aside 20 minutes a day to go back through some of the content in this book.

As you do, think about what you're currently doing and ask yourself if it's in line with the bigger picture. It may help you shake some of your monkeys when you put all of the information together. Our bodies are complex machines and require multiple things to happen in order for us to be at optimal health, and in turn, achieve optimal weight loss.

My Wish for You

I've seen so many transformations of spirit. As the weight comes off and your health comes back, it becomes easier to love yourself. I hear the joy in your voices and see it in your posts on my community on Facebook. How many of you feel the change at the deepest level of your being?

For those who have yet to experience these changes, it's coming.

My wish for you is to love yourself again, or for the first time. The most important relationship you'll ever have is the one you have with yourself.

I love my husband, family, and friends and will always go to the mats for any of them. But it wasn't until I went to the mats for myself that I realized how much more important that was. Loving myself, fighting for myself, changed every relationship I have and had.

The good relationships just got so much better and the toxic ones were left behind. I just keep thinking about what Glinda, the good witch, said to Dorothy, "You've always had the power my dear, you just had to learn it for yourself."

That sums it up perfectly.

What's Next?

One last thing, if you aren't already doing so, I suggest you pop onto Facebook and go to the public It Starts With The Food page to see what I'm posting. You can make it part of the 20 minutes since some of the emails are quick reads. I'm not asking you to read each and every article I post, but they are relevant to our lifestyle and contain information you will find relevant.

Take the time to fill your toolbox with information that will help you succeed and reach your goals, you're worth it.

Working Together

We have new members joining our Facebook page every day. Our group is becoming the pebble in the pond, creating a tidal wave of awareness. Most, if not all, of us have been searching for a way of life that allows us to have health, a weight we can be happy with, and ultimately the freedom to enjoy our lives.

I want you all to keep in mind, as we all go on this journey together, that what we do and the changes we make to our lives is knowledge gained… and we get the privilege to then pass it on to others.

I encourage you all to be fully present during this time: take note of things that work for you, things that might not work, and share them with me so I can pass it onto the group.

I'm one person, with my own very individual experience. The beauty of working together is we get to share these experiences and help each other.

Ultimately, this whole life thing is a series of connections with others.

The way for us to get out of it with happiness and an ounce of sanity left, is to do it together. Okay, I'm putting pom-poms down now.

Visit me at ItStartsWithTheFood.com **and sign up for my weekly newsletter which includes new recipes, rants and more or join a** Nourish, Grow & Thrive 3- or 6-Month Coaching Package **for even more support, community, and discounted 1:1 coaching packages.**

About the Author

Heather Parker is a Ketogenic Lifestyle coach living in Central Florida with her husband, daughter, two boys, and a mess of pets. Heather spent most of her life battling health problems and weight fluctuations before she finally found ketogenics in May of 2014; Heather completely transformed her health by switching to a ketogenic lifestyle. Now, Heather wants to help other women (and men) who are stuck on the hamster wheel of conventional dieting to make the connection between their body, mind, and soul and to find their "happy."

Heather offers private coaching, as well as the Nourish, Grow & Thrive 3- and 6-Month Coaching Packages. She is also the author of a ketogenic recipe book, Kickin' It in the Kitchen, Ketogenic-Style.

You can contact Heather by emailing her at heather@itstartswiththefood.com or by visiting the It Starts With The Food Facebook page.

Appendix for Keto-Friendly Foods

Fats:

- Avocado
- Beef tallow
- Butter
- Chicken fat
- Ghee
- Lard
- Macadamia nuts
- Mayonnaise (watch out for added carbs)
- Olive oil
- Coconut oil
- Coconut butter

Protein:

- Fish - wild caught
- Shellfish
  - Clams
  - Oysters

- Lobster
  - Crab
  - Scallops
  - Mussels
  - Squid
- Whole eggs - organic, pasture raised
- Meat - look for grass-fed and finished
  - Beef
  - Veal
  - Goat
  - Lamb
  - Other wild game

Pork - look for humanely raised without nitrates of any kind

- Pork loin
- Pork chops and roasts

Poultry - organic, pasture raised

- Chicken
- Duck
- Quail
- Pheasant

Bacon and Sausage - sugar and nitrate-free

Vegetables:

- Alfalfa sprouts
- Any leafy green vegetable
- Asparagus
- Avocado
- Bamboo shoots
- Bean sprouts
- Beet greens
- Bell peppers
- Bok choy
- Broccoli
- Brussels sprouts
- Cabbage
- Carrots - use in limited quantity for soups and such
- Cauliflower
- Celery
- Celery root
- Chard
- Chives
- Collard greens
- Cucumbers
- Dandelion greens
- Dill pickles - organic (limit these due to high sodium content)
- Garlic
- Kale

- Leeks
- Lettuces and salad greens
  - Arugula
  - Boston lettuce
  - Chicory
  - Endive
  - Escarole
  - Fennel
  - Mache
  - Radicchio
  - Romaine
  - Sorrel
- Mushrooms
- Olives
- Onions
- Radishes
- Sauerkraut - watch for added sugar and choose organic
- Scallions
- Shallots
- Snow peas
- Spinach
- Sprouts
- Summer squash - limit to 1 cup due to higher carb count
- Swiss chard
- Tomatoes
- Turnips
- Water chestnuts

Dairy:

- Heavy whipping cream
- Full-fat sour cream – organic and grass-fed whenever possible
- Full-fat cottage cheese
- All hard and soft cheeses - 1 ounce is considered a portion
- Cream cheese - 1 ounce equals one portion
- Unsweetened whole milk yogurt - be very careful and look at labels! Grass-fed and organic. Carbs should be limited to no more than 6 grams per serving.

Nuts and Seeds:

Look for organic, raw and preferable soaked and sprouted. A serving of nuts is almost always ¼ cup.

Nuts:

- Best choices due to lowest carb count
  - Macadamias
  - Pecans
  - Almonds

- o   Walnuts
- Higher in carbs, so these should be limited
  - o   Cashews
  - o   Pistachios
  - o   Chestnuts
- Nut flours, such as almond flour and coconut flour

Seeds:

- Pumpkin
- Chia
- Flax
- Sunflower
- Sesame

Sweeteners:

- Stevia — I like Sweet Leaf brand because it doesn't contain maltodextrin
- Erythritol
- Xylitol

Fruits:

- Lemon
- Lime
- Raspberries - limit these to a handful as a treat
- Blueberries - limit these to a handful as a treat

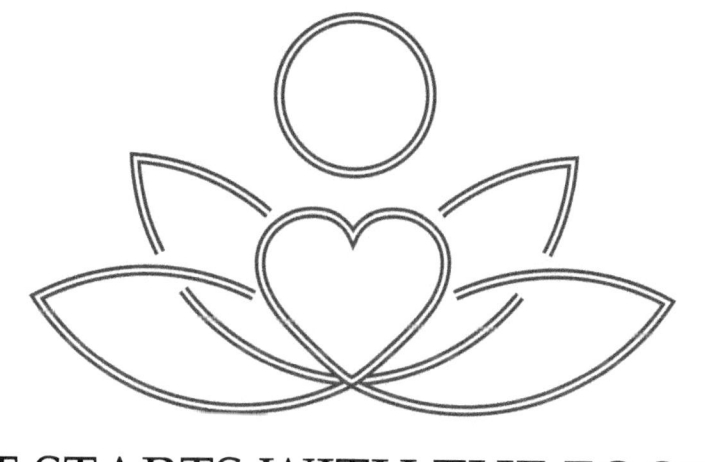

IT STARTS WITH THE FOOD